STRETCHING

FLEXIBILITY EXERCISES FOR THE TOP TEN ACTIVITIES OF ACTIVE PEOPLE OVER FIFTY

ALICIA DIAZ
LEE DAVIDSON

TABLE OF CONTENTS

Just For You!

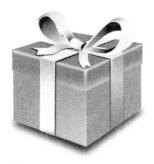

A FREE GIFT TO OUR READERS
Claim Your Gift At:

www.healthylifeafter50.com

INTRODUCTION

Life begins at 40, they say. But if you're doing it right, the real fun starts at 50. If physical aches, pains, and inflexibility don't plague you, that is.

Are you physically ready for what life at 50+ has to throw at you? There's more time to get recreational, there are possibly high-energy grandkids to keep up with, and then there's the opportunity to look your best now that you're no longer a slave to the corporate system. If you've just hit the big 5-0, or if you're hurtling there at great speed, or even if you're heading towards the next milestone in your life, there's no reason you should spend it with pain, discomfort, and declining health on your side.

It doesn't matter what stage you're at - you have every opportunity to turn your health around. There's a better version of life 50+ that awaits you! There's a version of life where you're physically fit; your body is melting fat at an appropriate rate (we all know round is a shape, but it's not *the* shape you're aiming for in your fun years), and you're able to keep up with the grandkids.

This version of life sees you hitting the tennis court (or golf course if that's more your speed), heading out for a gentle jog, lifting and carrying items on the heavier side of things, and strutting your stuff with confidence. After all, you're not aching, you're not straining, and you've got all the energy you need to live a healthy, fit and active lifestyle.

This version of life at 50 looks great, and that's because it is! You might be somebody's grandad or grandma, but that doesn't mean you have to surrender to the clutches of old age. That's not even a thing, really – *old age* is a state of mind. Why do we say that? Because how you look after your body determines how it responds, feels, and thrives. How you think and feel about yourself also plays a role in how young you are, regardless of the number attached to your age.

This brings us to the topic of *stretching* and its role in securing you the type of 50+ lifestyle you're interested in and *want*. Some 50+ folk who have discovered the effectiveness of stretching might even consider it the secret to staying fit, young, flexible, and healthy – and we're talking about mental health and fitness too.

Before we continue, you're bound to be wondering why the heck you should listen to us. Who are we, and what makes us authoritative figures on the topic of health, fitness, and 50+ living? Well, that's where it gets interesting. We are a duo who come from your neck of the woods – age-wise, that is.

We are Alicia Diaz & Lee Davidson, and we like to think of ourselves as a formidable duo in doing this *50+ life thing*. We're not some 30-somethings trying to sell you a book because we know a little something about fitness and the aging human form. Just like you, we have breached the border of 50, and we're well on our way to the next milestone.

In our 20s, we were *those* types. You know the types that like to hit the tennis court on a Tuesday evening and head out for a Sunday morning run? We were the type of people that planned our vacations around what sporting facilities were available. We were probably called "fitness freaks" or sports junkies by our neighbors. Yup, we were those people.

And then it happened.

Kids.

As you may well know, athletics and just about everything else that makes you uniquely you, takes a proverbial back seat when the kids come along. And before you know it, you've reached 50, the kids have bid you a fond farewell to live their happy lives without you (well mostly - and sob!), and you're stuck there with your aged form, lack of flexibility, and a "what now" black cloud hanging gloomily over your head.

 We were empty-nesters, and we were unfit. What an unattractive combination – for us at least!

We could have let it get us down and settle into "getting old," but we didn't. Instead, we started to relive our youth and enjoy all the things we left behind. As they say, "it's like riding a bicycle." It all came hurtling back at us. Our passion for being active was alive again, and we were ready to get back on that bike! Since we have, we've connected with more like-minded 50+ers than we can remember, all looking to do the very same thing but without the know-how to get started.

And that's where we come in.

We don't just want to help other people in their 50s reach their fitness goals and get strong and active again – we have a *passion for it*. And this book serves to help you and others who want to pick up where they left off in their youth and get going again. In short, if this sounds like you – this book is for you!

If you're a little pensive about getting started, don't worry! This isn't about overwhelming you with exercises, rules, and regulations that make your life uncomfortable and scare you witless. In the pages of this book, we will focus on various facets of stretching and how you can incorporate it into your life naturally and healthily.

We will discuss staying strong after 50, the benefits of stretching, and how to get started (and keep going).

Life is amazing after 50, especially if you're physically able to enjoy it. Don't take our word for it, though – learn everything there is to know in this book and see for yourself.

Alicia Diaz | Lee Davidson

AGING & FLEXIBILITY

Before we leap into how the body ages and what that does to flexibility, let's consider why stretching is essential. We'd like to start by saying that stretching isn't only essential to people in the 50+ club – it's vital to people of all ages.

Most 50+ers think of fitness and immediately balk at the idea. They envision hours spent on the treadmill or struggling under the weight of hefty dumbbells and bars. What we've learned in our mission to get fit and active after 50 is that there's an entirely different component of fitness that's just as important as getting your heart rate up and flexing those muscles – and it's called *stretching*.

If you think about it, you probably stretch every day. You may extend your arms and legs and breathe deeply when you get out of bed in the morning, or perhaps you even find yourself stretching out your back when you get up out of a chair. Stretching is a fairly natural thing to do, and if you learn how to hone your stretching skills and develop routines and activities that put stretching to good use, you can reap the physical rewards.

You can find yourself squatting down to pick things up, easily stooping to catch your running grandchild, stretching up to reach distant objects and soon becoming more involved in the physical activities you used to enjoy in your youth. And you will do this while other 50+ers stare on, wondering what your secret is.

One of the inspirations for writing our series of *Life After 50* books was a dear friend of ours who suffered an injury from doing something anyone of us could find ourselves doing. She was embarking on a flight and reached up from the seat to turn on the fan. And that's when it happened. The muscles in her rotator cuff tore, and she was faced with months of physical therapy just to ease the pain and lure her shoulder into enjoying a full range of motion once more. The sad part was that *this* friend of ours was once a very fit and active person – but in her youth.

You have to understand that it wasn't her *age* that caused the injury but rather a combination of becoming less and less active as she aged. Just like us, she had allowed physical exercise to take a back seat while she focused on raising a family. While she probably didn't notice it happening at the time, each year that passed, her muscles and tendons tightened and stiffened just a little more. We understand it was a rather rude awakening for her, especially knowing that a simple routine of daily or weekly stretching could have guaranteed an entirely different outcome. By that, we mean she would have stretched up to turn on the fan, and that would have been the end of that – no pain, no injury, and no months of physical therapy. Let's quickly look at the benefits of stretching before we move on.

Direct Benefits of Stretching

Relaxation. Stretching isn't purely functional; it also feels great! According to Healthline, stretching can release endorphins in the body. These endorphins are responsible for a whole host of feel-good things happening in the body. For starters, they reduce pain and elevate the mood. Then, they also relieve muscle tension, bust stress, and increase both blood circulation and flexibility while improving your posture. The more often you stretch, the more your body enjoys all of these endorphin-inspired benefits.

Flexibility Improvement. Stretching increases flexibility by lengthening the muscles and improving posture. This is the very reason why most personal trainers will insist on stretching before and after exercise. Increasing your flexibility won't just enable you to reach further than you have before (hey, you might even find yourself easily touching your toes sans grunting and groaning!). It also ensures that strenuous activities don't result in muscle injuries and strains. Stretching also promotes the longevity of your full range of motion – something that naturally declines as you get older and start moving a lot less.

Eliminates Pain. Aches and pains seem to come standard when reaching 50 and beyond. Just spend a while with a group of 50+ers, and once the chatting about the grandkids comes to an end, the conversation takes a dip to more sinister things, like pain in the lower back, neck, legs, shoulders, and arms. You may not already know this, but a lot of the pain we feel in our muscles is due to lactic acid buildup. In young people, it usually builds up when they do strenuous exercise. In older inactive people, it can build up when you do an activity, like carrying a few boxes, that's outside of the daily norm. Unfortunately, only a few 50+ers know that a bit of daily stretching can obliterate those pains! Stretching brings a fresh supply of oxygen to the muscles, reducing lactic acid production and eliminating any built-up lactic acid.

Improvement of Circulation. Stretching, although it's nowhere near as energetic as cardio, actually gets the blood pumping. As the blood flow increases, something else is happening in the body – oxygen levels start to rise, delivering much-needed nutrients to your muscles. At the same time, the process is working hard to remove metabolic waste from the body. If you're wondering what metabolic waste is, think uric acid, ammonia, and carbon dioxide. With all the extra blood flow and oxygen making their way to the muscles, you can expect reduced muscle stiffness and minimal recovery time. In fact, you can expect to bid a fond farewell to everyday muscle soreness!

These are just four of the many benefits of stretching, and you're about to learn a whole lot more about that! Before we move on, we'd like to introduce an interesting concept to you. The concept is that the human body was designed to move, always.

YOU WERE BORN TO MOVE, SO DON'T SLOW DOWN!

We've given this concept a lot of thought. As babies, we're born semi-helpless, but over the years, it becomes evident that we are born to move more and more and, at the same time, develop from strength to strength. If we said to you, "you are born to move," you might wonder what on earth we mean by that. It sounds simple, but it's easy to misunderstand the actual meaning behind it.

Way back in 1687, Sir Isaac Newton published his physical laws of motion and even though it's an age-old concept, they are innately true today. What are the core principles of Newton's laws of motion? The main principle states that inanimate objects at rest remain at rest unless an external force acts on them. Suppose you can imagine placing a rock on the ground. Once you've put that rock down, it follows Newton's laws of motion – it does not move.

The good news is that, as humans, we aren't rocks. Newton's law doesn't bind us. We are born to move and don't have to wait for an external force to come along to move us. We have a set of articulating joints and muscles and a central nervous system and brain that controls it all. Movement comes naturally to us.

The human body is a highly adaptable piece of equipment. If you start spending more time on the couch than being fit and active, you will adjust to that lifestyle. It may get quite comfortable relaxing on the couch - so you can't expect it to perform when you need to do some-thing slightly more active. Much the same, the body can adjust to increased levels of activity and fitness.

Here's what happens to the human body when we don't move enough:

- Reduced lung capacity
- Dwindling, weaker muscles
- Reduced bone capacity and an increased risk of osteoporosis
- Weight gain and a slower metabolism to match
- Reduced range of motion
- Weakened immune system (more illness and slow-down healing)
- Reduced cognition (and diminished brain function)
- An accelerated rate of aging (yikes)

According to recent statistics, as a society, we have stopped moving. In a report by the *International Council of Sport Science and Physical Education,* which you can read here: https://www.icsspe.org/ bookshop/designed-move, it states the following:

"In less than two generations, physical activity has dropped by 32% in the USA and 20% in the United Kingdom. In China, the drop is 45% in less than one generation. Vehicles, machines, and technology now do our moving for us. What we do in our leisure time doesn't even come close to making up for what we've lost."

Of course, a large part of the global population's movement decline is owed to televisions, mobile devices and other connected gadgets. Gone are the days when people believed that physical activity was a good way to pass the time. And then, before you know it, you're knocking on 50's door, and you've almost forgotten what it feels like to hold a tennis racket, wear a pair of running shoes, or swing a golf club. And even if you want to do these things, you avoid it because your muscle flexibility just isn't what it used to be, and you're scared of injury and pain.

With less movement and increasing age, energy levels decline, genetic and environmental factors take their toll, and aging muscles begin to lose mass, strength and flexibility. Everyday activities take more effort and result in more pain. In short, moving hurts.

Muscle Mass and Flexibility do a Disappearing Act

If you're already ensconced in the 50+ club, and you're not feeling as strong and spry as you once did, it's not all that surprising. As it turns out, just like bone density goes into decline as we age, so does muscle mass. Sarcopenia is the natural process of declining skeletal muscle as the body ages. After the age of 30, muscles start to decline at a rate of 3% to 5% each decade. Muscle loss doesn't just mean that you no longer look buff in a vest or can't quite manage a few heavy bags of groceries on your own anymore. It also increases your chances of fall accidents, getting low trauma fractures and suffering muscle strain when doing something seemingly effortless, like carrying a chair for someone.

Here's a newsflash! There's no gun to your head, and you are not forced to sit back and let the ravages of sarcopenia detract from your overall strength *and* life enjoyment. The secret is in keeping active. But don't take our word for it.

Dr Leython Williams, who just happens to be a licensed physical therapist specializing in musculoskeletal function and rehabilitation, says it best in one of his recent quotes on the topic. "As our bodies get older, we lose a small amount of flexibility as a result of the normal aging process. There is a loss of water in our tissues and intervertebral discs, increased stiffness in our joints, and a loss of elasticity in muscles and tendons. In our 20s and 30s, we must develop a consistent static and dynamic stretching regimen to establish and maintain flexibility and range of motion more easily into our older years."

We also like what Dr Rachel Reed, PhD, Pure Barre's manager of training development and barre kinesiologist says about flexibility and muscle mass as you age. She says, "Peak flexibility age for adults can differ from person to person and depends largely on their physical activity habits." She has also stated, "Notably, flexibility can be improved at any age when flexibility training is incorporated into a regular exercise routine. Adults need to be strategic about including flexibility training into their workouts because maintaining flexibility and physical function as we move into middle and older adulthood is associated with better quality of life and independent living."

Where to Start? It's All About Stretching

So, where do you start if you want to encourage more flexibility in your body? It all starts with two primary types of stretching.

- **Dynamic Stretching** This is where you repeat particular movements/exercises/stretches several times in a row. Think about doing four sets of ten squats – this is dynamic stretching.
- **Static Stretching** This is when you hold a particular movement or stretch for an extended period of time (usually 10 to 30 seconds), such as in the case of doing planks.

You don't have to worry about understanding these types of stretches too deeply right now - we cover these types of stretches in a bit more detail in chapter four.

The idea behind both of these stretches is to increase muscle flexibility and strength. When you first start stretching, it's bound to feel stiff and unnatural. You may start to think that you *can't* do it because your muscles seem to be fighting back. But the best advice we can give you is to persist.

With static stretching, the objective is to keep your muscle under tension for a specific period and then to increase the amount of time under tension as you progress.

For instance, when you start, you may only be able to hold a stretch for 15 seconds, but you should aim to increase that stretch hold to around 25 seconds in a few days. As your muscles become familiar with the movement and your flexibility gradually increases, you will find that you can do deeper stretches for longer. You may even feel that your muscle strength is developing too. It really does get easier the more you do it.

On the other hand, dynamic stretching is ideal for people who spend a large part of their day sitting down. The repetitive motion increases blood flow to soft tissues, reducing the risk of injury when making a sudden movement or reaching out for something (such as in the case of our friend with her rotator cuff injury). This type of stretching is also great for increasing your range of motion, which is something most 50+ers are interested in doing.

You're probably wondering how much time you have to spend stretching every day. Don't worry; we're not going to enroll you in hours of workouts and strenuous exercise. In fact, we have compiled several quick and easy five, ten, and fifteen-minute stretch routines for you to follow in chapter seven. They're perfect for doing first thing in the morning before you start your day to increase energy levels, ready your muscles for movement and reduce your chances of an injury.

YOUR CHOICES AND JOINT PAIN

As teenagers, it's drummed into our heads that the choices we make will have an impact on the rest of our lives. But somewhere along the line, we forget this lesson as adults. We stop thinking about actions and consequences when in reality, all the choices you make when you're heading towards 50 and breaching that border will have an impact on your quality of life going forward.

For instance, every time you turn down walking the dog or going to play tennis with your family, you're not just choosing a sedentary life-style (which you are); you're speeding up the process of aging. You're also losing out on the opportunity to stretch and strengthen muscles to reduce pain, and, of course, you're giving in to the ravages of stiffness and inflexibility. What you choose to do and *not* do will impact how quickly you age and what symptoms you welcome into your life. We often hear of 50+ers making one particular poor choice when they choose to head to a popular amusement park (we won't name names) in the Midwest, United States.

As it turns out, fall and spring are peak seasons for the 50+ crowd. 50+ers head to the park in droves, and one of the first things they do is hire a scooter to drive themselves around the park – it is hilly, after all. Walking those hills and going on the rides would be a *good* choice for them, yet most of them are there for the food, often high in empty calories and almost always deep-fried and topped with sugar. They're also there for a spot of shopping and watching a few shows, but physical activity? Certainly not. This is a lifestyle choice that will take its toll on *any* 50+er. Of course, you don't have to head to an amusement park to make a poor lifestyle decision – you can make poor lifestyle decisions in many other ways. Other poor decisions that come with physical consequences include:

- Eating processed foods because they're "quick and convenient."
- Avoiding daily walks because you're tired and achy.
- Saying you can't look after the grandkids because they're too active and you can't keep up.
- Choosing to drive to the store when it's just a few hundred meters away.
- Spending all day on the sofa because you're no longer working and don't have much to do.
- Never exploring gardening as a hobby because it requires bending, kneeling, stretching, and carrying things.

Do you see where we're going with this? All of these choices you think you are making for your health to avoid possible aches and pains can lead to *more* aches and pains in the long run.

Then there are those who have found the secret to living life young at heart and physically fit and active. These are *our* people, and we hope that you will join us. We choose to approach life with *movement as a priority*. We choose to play active roles in our grandchildren's lives – in fact, their energy levels have helped us get a bit fitter too!

We opt for playing at least one recreational sport a week and focus on stretching and doing strength training each day, even if it's just for a few minutes. We walk when we can, and we actively seek out hobbies that get us off the sofa and interacting with other 50+ers (and family members too).

WHEN GENUINE ACHES & PAINS COME TO PLAY

But what if you've got genuine joint pain to deal with? We knew this question would come up and we're prepared for it. The statistics tell us that many people over 50 have weight gain to blame for joint pain and stiffness. But there are also those, around 50%, who have some level of joint pain from the likes of Osteoarthritis, which is the most common form of arthritis. This condition results from cartilage deterioration. No one can really blame you for starting to think that you should move less to avoid the pain of bones rubbing against each other while exercising. The opposite is actually true, though.

While it's difficult to rebuild cartilage, it's good to know that some people enjoy 100% comfort while moving and exercising with no cartilage at all! The undeniable truth is that stretching lubricates joints and enhances and maintains a range of motion. This means that when you have joint aches and pains, stretching exercises *help*. There are several ways to thwart Osteoarthritis pain, by the way. Let's consider a few of those ways below:

Lose Weight. If you want to be kind to your joints suffering arthritis, be willing to take a load off them. How? By losing weight! Losing 10 pounds of weight can reduce around 40 pounds of pressure from your knees, for instance. That means that you reduce 4 pounds of pressure from your body for every pound of weight you lose. Also, you don't have to run marathons to lose weight when you're 50+. Making healthy food choices, walking the dog or walking to the store, and indulging in several stretching and possibly even strength training exercises each week should help you shed a few pounds the healthy way.

Get Fit! Most people don't know this, but there's a difference between losing weight and getting fit. You can shed 30 pounds of weight through dieting but still be weak with dwindling muscle mass and inflexibility. Getting fit strengthens the joints and supporting muscles as well as protects the full range of motion. You don't have to go on a high impact run or join boot camp! Instead, look for low impact exercises, such as daily stretching, swimming, cycling, walking, or doing a low-tempo circuit at the gym.

Say No to Sugar. Sugar finds its way into almost everything. It's in sodas, biscuits, and even in "healthy" breakfast cereals. We also tend to pop a spoonful of it into our tea or coffee, inadvertently drink it in fruit juice and spoil ourselves to sugar-laden treats whenever they're available. Why not, right? You're 50+ and you deserve to enjoy life's pleasures. Well, the problem with sugar is that it exacerbates arthritis pain. Consuming excess sugar will cause your body to release cytokines, which are pro-inflammatory proteins. Once they're in full swing in your body, they exacerbate any inflammatory conditions you have. If you have arthritis, cytokines will make it worse. Reducing your sugar intake will make a big difference to the amount of stiffness, pain, and swelling you experience.

Eat More Fresh Fruits and Veggies & Reduce Red Meat. Low calorie and nutrient-dense foods are the best choices for 50+ers with arthritis. In fact, studies have found that an increased intake of fresh fruits and veggies can lead to lower levels of inflammation. Of course, you know that arthritis is inflammatory, so eating for an anti-inflammatory effect can be most helpful. Unfortunately, and we know this is tough news to accept for many 50+ers, red meat has been linked to increased inflammatory markers such as interleukin-6, homocysteine, and C-reactive protein. If you're living on red meat and fries, it's time to reconsider your diet. Fresh fruits and veggies that are best for fighting the aches and pains of inflammation include garlic, ginger, broccoli, kale, spinach, berries, and grapes, to name a few. You don't have to start turning every meal into a medley of veg, but opt for oats and fresh fruit for breakfast and possibly even light coconut oil stir-fry veggies for dinner. You can mix it up without eating a bland diet.

Get Enough Sleep. Aim for at least seven hours of sleep per night. Sleeping enough each night gives your body sufficient time to rest and repair. Managing arthritis effectively requires a decent amount of sleep, but the pain alone can often result in a lack of sleep. The good news is that a few muscle stress-relieving stretches can help ease your muscles into rest mode.

Quit Smoking. Unfortunately, smoking is linked to increased arthritis pain. Researchers have been unable to explain exactly why, but they suspect it sparks a faulty immune system functioning, especially in people who are predisposed to getting arthritis. Lung capacity is also greatly reduced when smoking, and we all know how important it is for the body to get a decent supply of oxygen to all the cells for repair and recovery. By quitting smoking and then participating in stretching to increase lung capacity, you can help your body heal arthritic aches and pains a lot quicker.

THINGS JUST DON'T MOVE LIKE THEY USED TO

Experiencing a reduced range of motion is often the first tell-tale sign of being inactive when aging. If you find that you just can't move your joints in all the directions they could move in before; you're a victim of diminished ROM (range of motion).

Each joint in the body has an established "normal" range of motion, and as you age, this reduces considerably. Let's rephrase that. This reduces *considerably* if you're not consistently making use of that range of motion. Taking the time to move your joints through their full range of motion regularly is vital to aging with a healthy range of motion intact.

If you're anything like we were a few years ago, you'd be empty nesters who had become increasingly inactive over the years. And when the nest emptied, and you stood there feeling a sense of loss as you waved goodbye to your kids on their new adventures, you were probably well aware that all the joints and muscles in your body no longer move as they used to some twenty-odd years ago.

 Things have stiffened, seized, and become inflexible – you're almost expecting to hear squeaking and scraping as you move around.

Here's some good news for you! Even if you have already lost some of your range of motion, you can reverse the effects by actively starting stretching and flexibility training. So not only does stretching maintain (and protect) the range of motion – it can also reverse a poor range of motion too! This news alone was enough to get us started.

SCIATICA PAYS YOU A VISIT

Sciatica is a painful disorder that affects many people over 65 worldwide. The worst part of sciatica is that it can come on suddenly like a thief in the night, or it can gradually work its way into your life over time. Some describe sciatica as a burning sensation that hits them square in the back and then shoots down the back of both legs or even just one leg. It doesn't sound like fun, and it really isn't. Sciatica is caused by inflammation and irritation of the sciatic nerve in the back.

The main symptom of sciatica is pain, and it's not just pain in the back and legs. Some 50+ers with sciatica complain that even their hips hurt when they sit down. People cannot move their feet or lower legs in more advanced cases without experiencing severe searing pain. While sciatica almost always affects only one side of the body, the entire body is negatively impacted because of the debilitating pain it causes. What makes sciatica a given or makes an existing condition worse is:

- Being overweight
- Lack of movement or no exercise (here's where some stretching can play a good role in sciatica management)
- Incorrect sleeping environment (it might be the mattress)
- Poor quality sleep

At this point, you've probably absorbed all the above information and wonder where you are on the spectrum of healthy or unhealthy. Are you making lifestyle choices that exacerbate the symptoms of aging? To help you better understand how much work you need to put in, we have created this quick self-evaluation test. Be honest with yourself while completing this survey.

A SELF-EVALUATION OF YOUR HEALTH

Scenario	Yes	No
I drink at least 4 to 6 glasses of water per day	2	1
I eat a selection of protein, veggies, and fruit daily	2	1
I stretch at least 3 times per day	2	1
I drink soda, sugary fruit juice, or alcohol daily	1	2
I need help carrying my groceries	1	2
My grandkids tire me out	1	2
I often have unexplained aches and pains	1	2
I participate in an active sport or hobby	2	1
I often lack energy to do daily chores	1	2
I am overweight	1	2
People always think I'm older than I am	1	2
I am happy with my physical appearance	2	1
Total		

Figure 0-1. Self-Evaluation

If you scored under 18, there's plenty of room for improvement. The main objective is to score 24. If you did this test and see room for improvement, you're in just the right place to get started.

What's the next step?

Paging over to Chapter Two: *The Upside of Stretching* is the very next step you need to take!

THE UPSIDE OF STRETCHING

One of the things we have come to terms with in life is that not everything is beneficial. It might have taken us 50+ years to figure this one out, but at least we're onto something good.

As you reach 50 and head beyond its borders, you will be inundated with tricks, hacks, and methodologies for extending your youth, tricking the clock, and looking your best. These present themselves on social media platforms, via text messages from friends who got them from friends (and their friends and so on) and even television adverts. One of the things we couldn't help, but notice was that so many of the marketing ploys (and that's exactly what they are, by the way) aimed at *us* were/are focused on shortcuts and value-less approaches. Heck, we even encountered a cream made from snail slime that claims to reverse the signs of aging in people 50 and above.

It's time for one of those reality checks. Not everything you encounter offering the secret (or path) to eternal youth and agility is truthful. In fact, many of them lack value. If someone (or an advert) tells you that it's the quickest and easiest way to weight loss, smooth, wrinkle-free skin, a placated bowel (as opposed to an irritable one), and gleaming muscles bulging in areas they never bulged before in your youth, you're being lied to. You're merely a money source for whoever is behind those empty promises.

What works? Hard work, works. Time and effort works. Stretching works. Because it is beneficial to you, it won't be a walk in the park. It will take some effort. So step away from fad 50+ers diet plans, stop buying those gimmicky "do this for 5 minutes a day" body transformation gadgets, and focus on something that's genuinely beneficial to you. The best place for anyone of our age to start is with stretching. In chapter one, we already covered the many benefits of stretching. Now it is time for us to discuss these benefits in a bit more detail.

One of the first things we need to mention is that it is essential to maintain a range of motion within your joints. If you don't, the muscles shorten and become tight – and trust us, that's uncomfortable. Remember that friend of ours who hurt her shoulder while reaching up from her seat on a flight? If you aren't willing to put in the effort now, that could be you. You could innocently reach up to say change a lightbulb, and all of a sudden, the pain and strain courses through your body, leading to months of rehabilitating treatments that rarely achieve the outcomes you hope for.

In short, stretching keeps your muscles healthy, strong, and flexible. Well stretched muscles are ready when you need them, and better yet, they're not prone to injury when you do need them. Stretching is a mere stepping-stone for more movement. So, if your goal is to become more active again, implementing a regular stretching routine should be your first step. But, of course, if you have any pre-existing conditions that have made exercise and stretching impossible over the years, it is best to consult with your physician before you start getting active.

What's the Big Deal About Stretching Anyway?

With all this talk of stretching, there's bound to be a few naysayers who have their doubts. You might wonder why stretching is important for someone over 50 when you seem to have gotten by just fine without it for all these years. The thing is, you have just got by. You haven't thrived, and we want you to thrive. You undoubtedly feel the niggling aches and pains that come with age, and the good news is that they are reversible. All hope is not lost! There's every reason why 50+ can be your best years yet. To give you something to go on, let's look at four targeted ways stretching can support active aging, and keep pesky muscle tightness and aches at bay.

Stretching relieves lower back pain and reduces symptoms of arthritis. Back pain has a way of sneaking up on us in our 50s. Lower back pain, in particular, is often the result of spinal stenosis, Osteoarthritis, or the one we all hate to admit, carrying extra weight. If you're extra sensitive to old age as some people are, the cartilage between the joints may degenerate and cause additional pain (this is actually stenosis). Osteoarthritis is also nothing to scoff at. It's a painful disease that affects 33% of 50+ers. While stretching cannot reverse the conditions affecting your lower back, it will go a long way to relieving the pain, improving flexibility, alleviating joint stiffness, and extending your range of motion. You could be bidding your back pain a fond farewell just by committing yourself to regular stretching.

Stretching reduces the risk of falling. Being 50+ can feel like warfare with the environment around you. Everything seems to want to knock you over, trip you up, or see you hurtling through the air. The reality is that it's not really old age to blame - it's your lack of balance and stability. While general imbalance comes with age, you can actually work on being more flexible, sturdy and balanced. Research shows that flexibility and range of motion are critical to creating the stability necessary to reduce the risk of falling. If you want to be a lot less wobbly on your feet, improving and retaining flexibility in the hamstrings and quadriceps is essential. These muscles directly impact your static balance. Another area that you need to keep mobile and strong are the hip joints because they also impact static balance. Before you ask, static balance is when you are standing still. On the other hand, dynamic balance is being able to maintain balance and be sturdy on your feet while you're moving.

Stretching strengthens the muscles, increases flexibility and improves range of motion – all things required for better balance. So long slip and fall incidents! You're soon going to be firmly planted on your feet!

Stretching supports good posture. Now that you're 50+, you have to pay for the sins of your youth. Don't worry; we're not going to dig too deeply into your past! One of the biggest consequences 50+ers pay is poor posture due to a life spent hunched over a desk, or worse yet, a mobile phone. Now, as a 50+er, suddenly you're sporting a hunched back or can only slump down in chairs. Now what? The very first thing you absolutely need to know is that poor posture compresses the spine, which in turn causes pesky lower back pain. With daily stretching, posture can improve, and pain can (and will) reduce. With regular and dedicated stretching (that's doing the *correct* stretches), you can significantly increase flexibility and loosen tight ligaments, muscles, and tendons.

Stretching improves energy and blood flow. While doing our research for this book, we came across some pretty interesting information on the role of blood flow (or circulation, as you might call it) on the body. For instance, did you know that having poor circulation can lead to lethargy, joint pain, hemorrhoids, poor mental clarity and even more severe conditions such as phlebitis, heart attacks and strokes? Blood flow also carries oxygen to all your vital organs, so if your blood flow is sluggish, the chances are that your organs aren't operating at their full potential.

Stretching is known to boost blood flow and send healthy oxygenated blood throughout the body. This leads to more energy, high-functioning organs, and less chance of falling victim to the conditions mentioned above. Stretches that help boost circulation includes arm swings, shoulder circles, lunges, leg swings, and squats. While stretching gets your circulation going, it also increases flexibility and increases range of motion – it's a great all-rounder!

STRETCHING TIPS & ADVICE

While we take a closer look at specific stretches you should focus on when you're 50+ in Chapter Six, we'd like to share a few tips and advice for safe stretching the right way below. Let's stretch!

Focus on major muscle groups. You should concentrate on stretching major muscle groups such as your calves, hips, lower back, thighs, neck, and shoulders. Ensure that you stretch each side of your body, focusing on stretching muscles and joints that you routinely use.

Don't bounce. For some reason, many people have an inner urge to bounce while stretching. Don't worry – we have all done it. Instead, stretch using a smooth movement, extending your muscles outward without bouncing. Bouncing may feel nice to start, but it's a surefire way to injure or strain your muscles. By avoiding bouncing, you ensure a smooth and gentle movement. If you feel any sharp pains while stretching, stop immediately.

Hold your stretch. Believe it or not, stretching is a slow and steady process. There's no race involved, so you're doing it wrong if you find yourself rushing through them. Instead, breathe normally and hold each stretch for about 20 to 30 seconds before moving on.

Don't aim for pain. Expect to feel tension while you're stretching, not pain. Stretching should feel good to your muscles, back, and joints. If stretching is painful, ease off to the point where you don't feel any pain, then hold the stretch. Sometimes a full stretch isn't possible, especially if you've been inactive for some time. Only stretch as far as you can without feeling pain until you've got more flexibility in the muscle. It develops over time – just be patient with yourself.

Once you start a stretching routine, keep it going. Like most things you try to do in life, you have to be consistent with stretching if you want to see long-term results. Stretching is something you have to do every single day. The more you stretch, the easier it will get. But, if you stop a few weeks in, you will find it challenging to get started again.

Know when to exercise caution. If you've got a chronic condition, an injury, or pain from a past injury, it's safe to say that you aren't going to stretch perfectly the first time around. It will take time and practice, and you might even need to learn variations of stretching techniques that cater to your specific physical ability and condition. However, that should not put you off. You should still consult with your physical therapist or a trainer to develop stretching techniques that work for you and your body. Also, be careful not to overdo it. Stretching doesn't mean you can't get injured.

Strive for balance. It's safe to say that at 50+, you won't suddenly achieve the balance of a 20-year-old. However, you can achieve equal flexibility and balance on each side. When stretching, focus on stretching each side equally. Focus on working towards feeling comfortable standing and moving through your stretches. Carry out each stretch slowly and with dedicated focus.

Use dynamic stretching for higher physical activity. If you're about to play tennis or do a boot camp workout, a dynamic warm-up is best. A dynamic warm-up is when you carry out movements similar to those used in your sport or physical activity. Dynamic stretches are done at a lower level than the actual activity. It simply prepares the muscles for what's to come.

HOW DOES STRETCHING WORK?

How does stretching actually work? Let's talk about the physiology of stretching. To put it simply, stretching involves the muscles and joints working together. By now, you are probably aware that tendons attach muscles to the bones. Muscles have the ability to make the body move by engaging the bones, tendons and ligaments. That said, the bones, tendons, and ligaments do not have the same ability as the muscles. Contraction and relaxation of the muscle adjust the tension on the joints, which leads to movement of the body. The idea of stretching is to make sure when the muscle, joints, tendons, etc., are performing work and contracting, the tension between them does not cause injury.

This very simplified explanation of how stretching works tells us that flexibility and range of motion rely on your muscles, cartilage and joints. When all of these are working together, you will notice a difference in your knees, ankles, and hips. They smoothly will bend further than before, extend more than ever, and be pain-free while doing so. One reason why it is crucial to stretch equally on both sides is that tired muscles will cause the opposing groups of muscles to work harder. You will see muscle fatigue on the other side of your body and the inability of the surrounding muscles to protect the joints from more severe injuries if your stretching is not equal on both sides.

IMPROVE YOUR QUALITY OF LIFE

Let's talk about your quality of life for a minute. Most 50+ers don't want to become a burden to those around them. They also don't want to spend every waking minute glued to the sofa because everything just seems like an overwhelming physical effort.

Unfortunately, you will be a burden or possibly immobile if you don't spend time keeping fit and active. Your energy and fitness levels aren't going to naturally improve as you get older. They will simply get worse. But by stepping in with some healthy stretching, you can interrupt the downward spiral of getting old and immobile. Stretching is not a quick fix, but it is the secret to a life of 50+ where you can bend and stretch for things easily, carry your own groceries, and endure fewer aches and pains along the way.

We talk from our own personal experience when we tell you that stretching makes you more stable, more able (to do so many things!), and more agile. Just a few years ago, we weren't playing the sports we love or heading out for a Sunday morning run. Everyday activities came with the risk of injury, and we dreaded the aches, pains and strains after a high-energy morning with the grandkids. All that has changed for us, and to be quite honest, it all started with a simple daily stretching routine.

We've already covered the benefits of starting your day with a few stretches, but it's a topic well worth revisiting. Before we move onto Chapter Three, let's recap all the ways in which you stand to benefit from a regular stretching routine.

The Benefits of Starting Your Day with Basic Stretches

1. Stretching kickstarts blood circulation, which activates the body and mind with a fresh flood of nutrients and oxygen. At the same time, muscles that have been at rest for many hours are slowly eased into activity. The boost of oxygenated blood will also give you a decent burst of energy for the day.
2. Stretching strengthens muscles and improves flexibility, which improves your posture, relaxes muscles, and warms them up.
3. Stretching gives back pain its marching orders! Stretching eases tension in the neck and back, helping to alleviate pain while strengthening the muscles at the same time.

A few years back, we might not have believed that our 50+ lives could look so different. Who knew that doing something as simple as stretching could change everything we expected in old age. And since we began introducing the concept of stretching to more 50+ers around us, we have seen significant improvements in their lives too. The challenge lies in getting started. You don't have to put in hours every day. You can focus on putting in just 20 minutes per day, four to five days a week. Keep this up for 21 days, and then decide what you think and feel. We're willing to bet you'll be hooked on stretching and revelling in the physical benefits. When we got started, we focused solely on carrying out a few stretches every morning and then every night before bed. After a few weeks, we both started noticing our undeniably increased energy levels, and so we decided to take it up a level (or three, actually). We started slow, but now we play sport, go for runs, keep up with the grandkids and have a newfound zest for life!

IT'S TIME TO STRETCH!

We've spoken quite enough about how stretching works, the benefits, and why you need to start today. Now, it's time to consider which stretches are best for you. To begin with, we have selected seven of the stretching exercises we thoroughly enjoyed when we first started stretching. We call these our quality of life stretches because they really did a great job of improving ours! If you ever get to meet us (wouldn't that be great!), you will quickly discover that we're a couple that likes to practice what we preach. Every exercise featured below is a routine that kickstarted our way back to health – and still use today.

To get you started on your journey, spend at least 10 minutes every morning practicing these simple stretch exercises shown in the next few pages.

KICKSTART YOUR FITNESS JOURNEY WITH
THESE 7 STRETCH EXERCISES

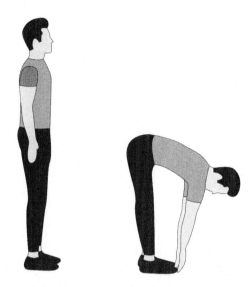

Figure 1-1. STANDING TOE TOUCH

1. Standing Toe Touch

- Stand up straight, look directly ahead with your feet shoulder-width apart and toes facing forward.
- Your starting position is standing with your arms extended down to your sides.
- Bend forward at the torso while keeping your arms out in front of you and your body relaxed. Then reach your fingers straight down toward your toes while bending your knees slightly.
- Hold that stance for just a few seconds and then return to the starting position. Repeat the same motion 10 times. Do not bounce.

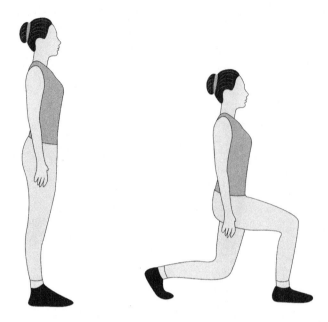

Figure 1-2. FORWARD LUNGE

2. Forward Lunge

- Stand upright, look directly ahead, with your feet shoulder-width apart. Your toes should be facing forward.
- Move your right leg forward to take a big step.
- Lower your body until your right thigh is parallel to the floor.
- Press your right heel to drive back up to the upright starting position.
- Repeat the same movement on the left side, then alternate each side 10 times.

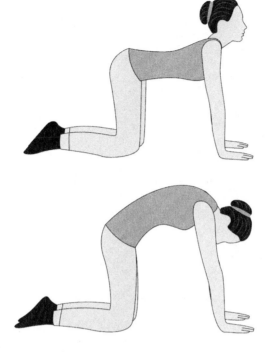

Figure 1-3. BACK ARCH STRETCH

3. Back Arch Stretch

- Start positioned on the floor with your hands and knees hip-width apart.
- Arch the back, drawing your belly button up toward your spine while keeping your hands at shoulder-width apart. Hold for a brief second.
- Slowly relax the muscles allowing the stomach to naturally fall toward the floor, while exhaling. Keep your shoulders and hips in the very same position.
- Return to the starting position and repeat this motion a total of 10 times.

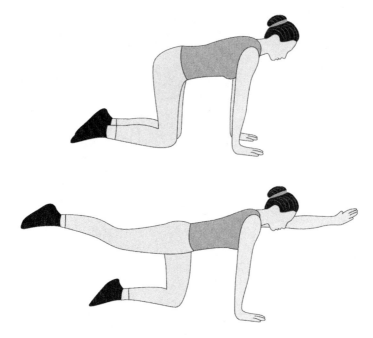

Figure 1-4. ARM & LEG EXTENSIONS

4. Arm & Leg Extensions

- Begin this exercise on your hands and knees - they must be positioned hip-width apart.
- Lift one hand and point the arm out straight in front of you. Then, extend the opposite leg behind you straight back. Keep your hips squared to the ground as you keep your weight centered.
- Keep your abs engaged throughout the entire motion.
- Hold for a few seconds, then return to the starting position.
- Repeat each side 10 times.
- If this is challenging at first, extend your arm and leg separately until you are stronger.

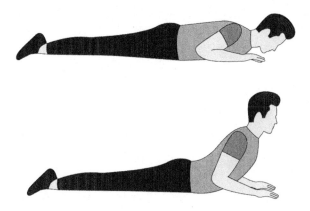

Figure 1-5. BACK EXTENSIONS

5. Back Extensions

- Lie down on the floor face down with your legs straight behind you.
- Put your elbows on the floor and place your hands just under your shoulders.
- While your hips continue to stay pressed on the floor, push your shoulders up and keep your head in a neutral position.
- Hold this stance for a few seconds, and then slowly lower yourself to the starting position.
- Repeat this motion 10 times.

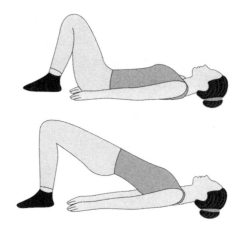

Figure 1-6. PELVIC LIFT

6. Pelvic Lift

- Lie down on your back while you bend your knees. Keep your feet flat on the floor. With your palms down, keep your arms close to your sides.
- Press down through your heels and lift your hips off the floor.
- Keeping your shoulders on the floor, lift your body until your hips make a straight line from your shoulders to your knees. Ensure your knees are lined up with your feet.
- Hold the bridge at the top for a few seconds before lowering back down. Repeat this motion 10 times.

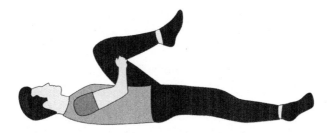

Figure 1-6. KNEE TO CHEST STRETCH

7. Knee to Chest Stretch

- Lie down facing the ceiling with both of your legs resting on the floor straight out ahead of you.
- Bring one knee up into your hands. Then pull your knee toward your chest.
- Hold for a few seconds and lower that same knee back down onto the floor in a resting position.
- Take a breath, then repeat the same steps with the other leg.
- Repeat 10 times for each leg.

Easy peasy, right?

The stretches above are some of the easiest you will come across. We recommend focusing on these first before trying any other stretching exercises featured later in this book. These exercises increase mobility, flexibility and range of motion and are perfect for absolute beginners getting back into fitness and active people who suffer from exercise-related aches and pains.

You will find that you are effectively stretching major muscle groups in all areas of the body by doing each of these stretches. Talk about a full-body workout! In addition to all of that, you will also find adding stretches to your daily routine provides opportunity for a few minutes of mindfulness each day. And we all know how beneficial mindfulness can be to mental and emotional health. Now, we're not saying that doing these simple stretches will see you drafted as a professional footballer or chosen to enter the Olympics as an agile 50+ gymnast. But they will get you back on your feet, free from pain, and feeling far more flexible than you have been in years. This could be the first step you take towards running, cycling, playing with the grandkids and getting things done around the home without living in fear of injury and pain. Without sounding too dramatic, this could be a monumental moment in your life (it was in ours): the day you decided to stretch!

Before we move on, we'd like to tell you about our friend, Paula. Paula is just like you and us in that she has breached 50 and finds herself retired (it's an entirely different lifestyle, isn't it?) Paula recently told us that she has just started realizing how much time she has for doing all the activities she wants now. Her excitement, which was reminiscent of a little kid's, was also the inspiration for us writing this book. We often fondly remember her telling us, "This is the first time of my life I haven't been in school, teaching school, or raising children to go to school since I was five years old! I almost don't know what to do with myself. Oh yes, I do. I'm going to go ride my bike!"

We want other 50+ers to be just as excited about older life as Paula is. If you're not excited for your 50+ life yet, get excited! Finally, you have the opportunity to enjoy unlimited fun! You don't have the same responsibilities that you used to, and now all you have to focus on is living life to the full! Add some stretching to your life, and you can do just that!

Next up on our list is Chapter Three: *Living Pain-Free Past Fifty*. This chapter focuses on the everyday aches and pains that 50+ers deal with and how something as simple as stretching can eliminate them from your life.

3

LIVING PAIN FREE PAST FIFTY

Most fellow 50+ers are absolutely gobsmacked when we tell them that nearly 50% of club members (that's the 50+ club, by the way) have creaking joints. By that, we mean that they have joint pain or some form of arthritis. This doesn't paint a rosy picture for the years to come, does it?

For us, it almost seemed like there was some sort of glitch in reality. You spend the majority of your 30s and 40s looking after children and putting them ahead of everything else, and then when you get to the so-called "golden years," you get the news that everything is about to start hurting, bending, breaking and just not functioning like it used to. It sounded more like cheap tin years than golden years to us! The idea of a frail and painful life ahead of us was just one of many motivating factors for getting us off the sofa and back into fitness.

There's no good reason why you have to be a statistic. Why do you think only 50% of 50+ers have these ailments? What are the other 50% doing? Ahh, nobody has ever really thought about that, have they? Most people hear that half the older community has aches and pains, and they just accept that they will be part of *that* 50% when their time comes. We're here to tell you to stop accepting an ill-advised fate because there's plenty you can do to push yourself into the other 50%. That's a statistic you *want* to be part of – the 50% that's not suffering arthritis, aches, pains, lethargy, and general disgruntlement at life. Of course, getting up and starting to move around actively and stretch is only *part* of the process. You also need to adjust your mindset, which means no more negative thinking about getting older and no more complacency (a perfect example of complacency is when you just accept that life's filled with aches and pains).

There's a rather interesting study that illustrates this point nicely. According to information published in the National Library of Medicine, a study was hosted in 2002 to research if longevity could increase by having a positive self-perception of aging. 660 participants, each of whom was 50 years and older, were assessed to determine whether they had a positive self-perception of aging or a negative one. The findings were ever-so interesting! The study found that 50+ers who had a positive mindset about aging and wanted to live their best life lived on average 7.5 years longer than those who had a negative mindset and approach. Wow! That's 7.5 years more time with your family and friends – that's a blessing! You can read more on the study here: https://pubmed.ncbi.nlm.nih.gov/12150226

When people in the over 50 age group have pain, they often overlook it and brush it aside, which leads to it becoming a chronic problem. 50+ers believe it's some sort of right of passage to put up with a chronic pain that is endless instead of taking action to reduce and possibly even end it.

ATTITUDE AND ACTIVITY

While we have already touched on both of these elements in the opening paragraphs of this chapter, it's important to reiterate: the only way to beat the negative effects of aging is to get active and adopt the right attitude/mindset. You can try a multitude of pills, tinctures, potions, creams, and pain killers, but none will be quite as effective as getting involved in physical activity and getting your mind thinking more positively about the next stage of life. You might be thinking that this is a tall order – in fact, two tall orders. How do you suddenly get active when you lack the motivation and have aches and pains plaguing your body? And how do you miraculously adopt a new mindset? These aren't easy asks; we get that. But if you look at attitude and activity from a new perspective, you might be inspired to take the first steps.

You see, mindset and activity go hand in hand. They're soul mates. When you're active, it naturally spurs on a more positive mindset. And when you think positively, it makes it easier to get active (or *want* to get active). And even more inspiring should be the news that exercise can change the brain to protect memory and thinking skills. We know how foggy our brains can get beyond 50! Who wouldn't want to boost a better memory and promote improved thinking skills?

According to a rather interesting article published by Harvard Medical School, any form of exercise that elevates the heart rate actually increases the size of the hippocampus. This is the very part of your brain that's responsible for learning and verbal memory. It's also the part responsible for the decline of clear thinking and memory as you get older. You can read more on the article here: https://www.health.harvard.edu/blog/regular-exercise-changes-brain-improve-memory-thinking-skills-201404097110

The Alzheimer's Society tells us that the number of people living with dementia worldwide is expected to double every 20 years. By 2050 it is projected there will be 115 million people with dementia worldwide, 71 per cent of whom will live in developing countries. Of course, you don't want to be part of the statistic in the lead up to 2050!

Everyday Pain

Below we share valuable insights on how stretching helps alleviate aches and pains and how it can genuinely prevent future aches and pains when done consistently and correctly. Pain is like a naughty spoiled brat that's never been disciplined. If you let it run wild and never put measures in place to reign in it, it will wreak havoc on your body. You will become a frail victim of decreased socialization, reduced mobility, slow rehab, and increased healthcare needs. And when you're suffering all of this and your quality time with family and friends is steadily declining, you're a prime candidate for depression and cognitive impairment. The effect of isolation on seniors in nursing homes during COVID-19 lockdowns is a fine example of the detrimental impact isolation and "going nowhere" can have on 50+ers. And that's just the mental aspects of everyday pain. The 50+ crowd is infamous for mismanaging their pain. Young people develop an ache and think, "Hey, that's not right. I must fix this immediately!" and older people think, "Another ache! I guess this is what getting old feels like" before returning to their sofa for a few more hours of sitting around. Do you see the problem with this picture? You should! The most common everyday aches and pains that 50+ers spend their time trying to ignore include:

- Stiffness in the hands, knees, and hips
- Dull aches in the wrist, thumb, and ankle joints
- Neck pain
- Shoulder and back pain
- Lower back pain
- Migraines (thanks to hormonal changes)
- Pain in the arms and legs

When aches and pains come along, there's usually a reason, and a vast majority of the time, there's a stretching regimen and positive thinking pattern that can rectify it. With that said, let's talk about the types of stretches that are ideal for those everyday aches and pains.

Stretching for Everyday Aches and Pains

Of course, you don't have to be an acrobat or even very flexible to use stretching to ease your aches and pains. Even if you feel like you're not bending, reaching, or stretching very far, something good is still happening within the muscles and joints of your body – it's rather therapeutic. Consistency is key! By that, we mean you cannot get excited about stretching and do it for a few days and then stop because you don't see instant results. You have to do a little bit every day, and we promise you that you will see the benefits with time.

Below is a brief list of rules we came up with for all 50+ers who want to start stretching to reduce pain in the body.

- Stretch to warm up
- Stretch to cool down
- Stretch at least once a day
- Wear something comfortable when stretching and exercising
- Extend into stretches slowly and never force it if your muscles feel tight
- Hold stretches for at least 30 seconds
- Breathe deeply and exhale slowly with each stretch
- Relax your body – don't stretch while in a stiff stance
- Stretch more than just the sore parts of your body
- Repeat every stretch without bouncing (one stretch is not enough)

Just like you gradually become better at mathematics as a kid because you practice it every day, your muscles will become more flexible and achieve more with daily practice. And yes, stretching can be a little painful. Never force a stretch if the pain is unbearable but don't stop stretching just because you can feel your muscles pulling – if you go slowly and gently, you will do just fine. Many 50+ers looking for gentle stretching exercises find value in Hatha Yoga, which is worth looking up. These extended muscle stretches build strength and go a long way toward decreasing fatigue, pain, and mental and physical stress. Each stretch that we teach in this book is designed to help someone with the challenges of a 50+ body. Each stretch ensures your muscles become stronger, longer, leaner, and more flexible. In the end, everyday activities become easier and less painful.

David Nolan, who happens to be a respected physical therapist at the Harvard-affiliated Massachusetts General Hospital, said, "A lot of people don't understand that stretching has to happen on a regular basis. It should be daily." You can read more on David Nolan and his stance on the importance of stretching here: https://tinyurl.com/j9rfn224

JOINT PAIN, MUSCLE FATIGUE, AND CRAMPING

While most people believe that muscle fatigue, joint pain, and cramping are all afflictions reserved for the VIPs of the 50+ club, that's just not true. These issues can crop up in anyone who chooses to live a sedentary lifestyle or is overweight for their body type.

Let's start by discussing muscle fatigue and pain. Most online resources will tell you that muscle fatigue is a sure sign of an injury, infection, disease, or another underlying health issue. It is described as either a steady dull ache or a deeper sharp pain. Some people experience muscle pain all over their body in various areas, and others have centralized pain in one place. It all comes down your physicality, what your body has been through over the years, and how active you currently are.

 Once you start getting active again, you're sure to feel muscle pain, but that pain's referred to as "good feeling pain."

This is when you've put your muscles through their paces. You will also be left feeling mighty good about yourself because you know you've done something good. It's not a negative pain. This is the type of pain we want you to become familiar with. If you're a little achy in your arms and thighs from all the heavy-lifting you did while gardening, that's not a bad thing! That's a good thing! It's a bad thing if you've been lifting things incorrectly and now have pain in your back and neck. If you're experiencing muscle pain in the legs and arms, we encourage you to carry more things in the garden because it's quite an enjoyable and effective workout. When you get muscle pain from exercise, there's no need to seek out medical help. In a few days, the pain will ease, and if you're consistently active, you will stop feeling pain after exercise.

Muscle pain from an injury is a different story, though. It hurts to move around, and there's no positive element to it. You haven't done something good for your body, and in all honestly, you should seek out medical care before it becomes a chronic condition. Stretching is often used to help muscles heal from an injury, but in most instances, there are specific stretches chosen for you by your physiotherapist, who has a better understanding of your condition.

Joint pain is another area of concern for 50+ers. Joint pains can irritate your hands and feet, knees, hips, and spine. It's hard to pin down the pain because it's quite elusive – it comes and goes as it pleases. This type of pain most often makes an unwanted arrival when you move suddenly, do something you haven't done in years, or overexert yourself.

 Joint pain is often described as a tight, achy, and sore feeling in the joint area.

It can cause a burning sensation in some people, and in others, it presents as popping or crackling in joints when they move. Most people who experience joint pain think it's a first-class ticket to a few weeks in bed or on the sofa doing as little as possible, but that's the opposite of what you should do. How so? Well, according to Amy Ashmore, PhD, who works as an exercise physiologist at the American Council of Exercise, stretching is helpful for people living with joint pain and arthritis. You can read more on the article here where she explains that stretching lubricates the joints and enhances range of motion (and also maintains it), which is exactly what 50+ers want and need: https://tinyurl.com/umsxumc

Most joint pain sufferers have joint aches and pains because they:

- Have a past injury
- Continue to use the joint even when it sends out sharp pains.
- Have arthritis
- Are overweight, bearing too much pressure on the muscles and joints
- Suffer poor health in the form of stress or depression
- Live a sedentary life, very rarely getting active or doing anything that requires the muscles and joints to work

Here's a look at three of the best stretches for common joint pains:

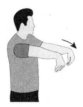

Figure 2-1 WRIST CIRCLES

1. Wrist Circles

- You can either sit or stand with this one.
- Keep your fingers straight, or allow them to curl into an unclenched fist naturally.
- Now rotate your hands at the wrist bone in circles to the left.
- Do this for ten rotations.
- Then stop and repeat the exercise, rotating your wrists to the right.

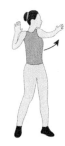

Figure 2-2 TORSO ROTATIONS

2. Torso Rotations

- Stand with your feet shoulder-width apart.
- Bend your knees slightly.
- Slowly and gently twist your upper body to the left while looking over your shoulder.
- Do not push too far.
- Hold that twisted stretch for 5 to 10 seconds.
- Repeat the stretch on the right side.

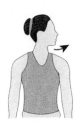

Figure 2-3 HEAD TURNS

3. Head Turns

- Start either sitting or standing
- Hold your head high and look directly ahead of you.
- Slowly turn your head to the right.
- Hold it for a second or two before returning to the center.
- Repeat this movement to the left side.
- Do a total of 10 repetitions.

The Importance of Stretching for Pesky Joint Aches & Pains

Your joint's range of motion is the biggest role player in how flexible and healthy your joint is. And what impacts your joint's range of motion? Your muscles! If your muscles elongate and become strong and flexible, your joint can move through its full range of motion without inspiring pain and inflammation. The amount of tension you have in the muscles surrounding a joint is critical to the joint's range of motion. If you have stiff and inflexible muscles, you won't be able to fully extend your legs up in the air while lying on your back (your knees will be slightly or very bent), or you'll struggle to touch your toes. To get your muscles stretched, elongated, and flexible, you need to ensure your posture is correct and that you do regular stretching exercises.

Stretching to Avoid Muscle Cramps

Muscle cramps are sneaking little things, aren't they? They suddenly arrive, and in an instant, you're left there clutching at your leg while your toes curl into unnatural positions, and your leg lifelessly locks into a weird trance. This is a good old-fashioned "Charlie Horse." At least that's what we've always called it. The best way to describe them is, Ouch! Muscle cramps are *not* comfortable.

Muscle cramps are involuntary contractions and can happen in the legs, back, and even the arms and hands. It's a spasm that eventually passes. It might not really feel like it in the very moment, but the best method of getting rid of these cramps is through massage (rubbing) and doing gentle stretches. Muscle cramps can also be a side effect of being short on magnesium, so if you often have cramps/spasms, you might want to look into taking a supplement.

Here are our top tips for giving a Charley Horse the boot and experience sweet relief:

- Drink enough water (and no, tea and coffee does not go toward your water intake)

- Eat food high in potassium and magnesium (or take a supplement)
- Stretch daily – when you wake up, before and after exercise, and when you've got nothing better to do
- Wear comfortable shoes that don't strain the muscles
- Limit your alcohol intake

If you've been relatively inactive for a long time, make gradual changes to ease your muscles into exercise and activity.

Stretching for Back & Spinal Pain

If you suffer from back and spinal pain and see a physician, they will present you with core and back muscle strengthening exercises to try out. Back and spinal pain is often a direct result of poor posture or using the incorrect methods to move heavy objects (and not so heavy objects, too).

When back muscles are well stretched and robust, they will be less prone to injury and strain. If your back has suffered a severe injury, follow your doctor's exercise and rehab program before getting into a strenuous activity again. In the next few pages we will recommend some back and spinal stretches for the 50+er.

The following exercises are meant to be performed slowly and steady to ensure the best results.

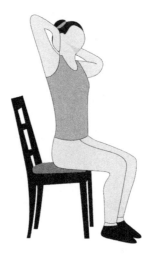

Figure 3-1 NECK STRETCH

1. Neck Stretch

This is good for easing spinal pain caused by the neck.

- Do this stretch while you are sitting on a firm chair. Keep your back straight and your feet flat on the floor. Raise your hands and place them behind your head with fingers interlocked as if basking in the sun on the beach.
- Slowly ease your head backward into your hands and lift your face towards the ceiling.
- Breathe in deeply. As you exhale, lean your left elbow down toward the ground and your right elbow up toward the ceiling.
- You should feel a gentle but supported stretch in your neck.
- Hold that position (which is only slight, by the way) for two deep breaths and then slowly return to the starting position.
- Repeat this on the opposite side. Try to do at least four reps on each side.

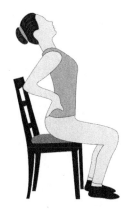

Figure 3-2 SEATED BACK BEND

2. Seated Back Bend

This stretch is good for the neck, spine, and back.

- Sit on a firm chair and position your feet flat on the floor with your back straight.
- Position your hands onto your lower back with fingers facing downward and thumbs wrapped onto your hips, pointing toward the front of your body.
- Push your hands into your hips/lower back and breathe in deeply.
- As you breathe out, push backward with your head and arch your back. Your chin should tilt upward, and your face should face the ceiling.
- Hold the arched position for the count of five deep breaths and then return to the starting position.
- Repeat this movement at least six times.

Chronic Pain and the Benefits of Stretching

If I tell you to think about chronic pain, conditions such as arthritis, lower back pain, and fibromyalgia probably come to mind. And what do most people do when they have pain? They seek out a pain killer. People head off to their local doctor (or call it in) to whine about the aches and pains they have been suffering for weeks, months, and years. Then, they spend the rest of their lives guzzling pills and taking it easy. And still, the pain persists, especially when the body gets used to the pain killers. According to ChoosePT, back in 2017 in the USA, over 191 million prescriptions were written for opioid pain killers. That's a jaw-dropping 58.7% prescription rate per 100 people. You can read up on this statistic here: https://tinyurl.com/7trwuftm

Most people don't realize that the only painkiller they need is daily stretching and that it's entirely free. Let's recap the benefits of stretching for pain:

- Increased pain tolerance
- Reduced weight for a slimmer you and less strain on muscles and joints
- Improved mood
- Stronger muscles and the ability to do more things for yourself (independence)
- Fewer aches and pains
- Improved flexibility
- Better sleep
- Improved circulation thus better functioning of organs and muscles
- Enhanced cognitive ability (no more foggy head)
- Increased energy
- More positive mindset towards aging

THE BENEFITS OF EATING WELL AT 50+

We couldn't really talk about living 50+ the healthy way without touching on diet, could we? And we know how sensitive people can be about their food and drink. We've often joked that you should never separate a man from his steak and beer or that women should be left to their decadent chocolate and red wine. But while this seems to be a societal norm, is it really a healthy way to be?

No, we aren't being one of "those" fitness couples that expect you to break up with all the good things in life and start measuring your food portions. But we are encouraging you to make *healthier* choices as often as you can. If you're in the habit of drinking red wine and eating chocolate daily, try to reduce that to three times a week instead. You'll still enjoy your favorite things, just without killing yourself in the process! You can also make small changes to the meals you eat. If you tend to like fried foods, look at the option of buying an air fryer, so you can still enjoy fried foods, except without the added oil and sodium. Being healthy is about being strategic, not about being overly strict or living a mundane life. We've already touched on making healthier food choices in the previous chapter, so we won't rattle on too much about it! We will say this though...

Now that you're expecting your body to perform, you have to feed your muscles (and brain) with nutritious food that has a healthy balance of protein, healthy fats, carbohydrates, fiber, vitamins, and minerals. Good nutrition comes with a world of benefits for us in the 50+ club. There's a reason why healthy diets are touted as a good thing from when we hit our teens to well into our golden years - because it's the truth! Here are a few of the reasons why you need to think about eating a healthy diet:

- Weight loss
- Lowered cholesterol levels
- Lower blood pressure
- Less risk of strokes, heart disease, and cancer

- Less chance of developing diabetes
- Stronger immune system (fewer pesky colds)

And when you pair a good diet with a decent amount of exercise, you're no longer a 50-year-old withering away. You're a strong independent man or woman in your own right. As you approach 60 and beyond, you will not have to fear losing your independence and needing to rely on other people just to do everyday things.

Here's a quick guide to boosting your diet:

Protein

According to Harvard Health Publishing, you should multiply your weight in pounds by .36 to determine how much protein you need per day in your older years. For instance, if you weigh 160 pounds, you should aim to get a minimum of 61 grams of protein per day (160 x .38 = 61). Getting the protein you need is easier than you think - there's no real need to revamp your entire shopping list. You don't have to eat like a bodybuilder just because you've started stretching.

You can have a cup of plain yogurt sprinkled with dry chia seeds and a handful of nuts on top for breakfast. For lunch, you can have a plain and simple peanut butter sandwich on wholewheat or brown bread. And for dinner, you can have a lean piece of salmon, baked potato, and salad. You're already well over 60 grams of protein. See how easy it is?

Carbohydrates

Everyone hears the word carbohydrates and wants to freak out. It's almost like we should be hauling carbs to the town square to be drawn and quartered while the rest of us watch on, shouting and jeering. Here's what most people don't know about carbs – they are an essential part of any diet. Carbs are your body's main source of energy. The energy from carbs fuels the central nervous system, kidneys, heart, and brain. Fiber is also a carbohydrate needed to maintain a healthy digestive system, leading to a lowered chance of heart disease and diabetes. Don't haul out the bags of crisps just yet, though - like with everything; moderation is key.

When it comes to getting enough carbs, it's best to follow the official Dietary Guidelines for Americans which states that carbohydrates should make up 45% of your daily calories. For example, if you eat 2,000 calories per day (which is in the range of normal), around 900 of those calories should be allotted to carbohydrates. Aiming for around 225 grams of carbs a day is good.

Healthy Fats

Another food type that's vilified is fat, but fat is good. There's healthy fat and unhealthy fat. To incorporate healthy fats in your diet, aim to eat avocado, walnuts, sunflower seeds, pumpkin seeds, chia seeds, fish, dark chocolate, olives, and plain yogurt. Easy to incorporate these into your diet, right? We think so!

Fiber

As you get older, the gastrointestinal tract can get a little sluggish. Many 50+ers experience uncomfortable IBS or just have such irregular systems that they're kept guessing. If you want to ensure that you don't suffer from constipation, high blood sugar, and high cholesterol levels, you need to welcome good quality healthy fiber to the party. Men over 50 need to consume 28 grams of fiber each day, while women should aim for 22.4 grams each day. Good fiber comes from fresh fruits and veggies, oats, legumes, beans, and lentils. If you haven't been getting much fiber, don't try to increase your intake suddenly. Easy does it. Slowly add a bit more fiber to your diet each week.

How do you get all the fiber you need? If you're eating your five fruit and veg a day, you're halfway there. Focus on sprinkling seeds, legumes, and beans onto your salads and side dishes. When you start thinking about it, it becomes an easy task.

Vitamins and minerals

The supplement industry's value was estimated at a jaw-dropping USD 140.36 billion in 2020. Its value is expected to rise over 151 billion in 2021. What does this tell us? It tells us that the vitamin and supplement industry has an exceptional marketing department that can sell anything to anyone, or the majority of the world population doesn't believe it's getting what it needs from the food they're eating. And perhaps everyone is eating that badly, but it really shouldn't be that way. If you focus on eating fresh whole foods and avoid buying convenience meals and processed meals, there's every reason to believe that you're getting most of your required vitamins from your food. Still, some people have deficiencies, and having a supplement isn't the worst idea. We recommend taking a good-quality multivitamin daily to cover the gaps that might be present in your diet. Other vitamins that 50+ers should ensure they're getting enough of include vitamin B12, D, and calcium. And, of course, for a strong immune system, zinc is needed.

Painful Inflammation & Eating for Anti-Inflammatory Effects

Painful inflammation is what you feel when your body is responding to toxins, infections, and injuries. As we get older, we're prone to painful inflammation. You might not know this, but certain foods and drinks you consume can play a role in flaring up inflammation. While you don't have to eliminate all these foods from your diet, you might want to reduce your intake to ease their effect on your body. Foods to avoid to reduce inflammation in the body:

- Processed meats
- Red meat
- Sugary drinks
- Alcoholic drinks
- Oily/fried foods
- Refined carbohydrates (this is white bread and white pasta)
- Dairy

Eating for an anti-inflammatory effect means eating foods that have a reputation for fighting inflammation. These include:

- Leafy greens (spinach and kale)
- Olive oil
- Almonds
- Fatty fish (tuna and salmon)
- Blueberries
- Brocolli
- Cherries
- Green tea

According to Dr. Welches, DO, PhD., a pain management specialist at Cleveland Clinic, anti-inflammatory eating doesn't mean you have to entirely cut out meat and dairy but reduce intake. He said, "A vegan or Mediterranean diet – or healthier eating inspired by these diets can control insulin levels, cholesterol levels, and reduce inflammation. The inflammation is the pain culprit."

An anti-inflammatory diet is a great pain killer and offers a whole host of other health benefits too. When you pair an anti-inflammatory diet with a decent stretch routine and stress management approach, you have a powerful tool at your disposal. This is certainly food for thought! Pun intended! You can read more on Dr. Welches anti-inflammatory eating information here: https://health.clevelandclinic. org/anti-inflammatory-diet-can-relieve-pain-age/

Diet Basics

As kids, we grew up learning what the food pyramid looks like. Unfortunately, the food pyramid we saw as kids is just not the one that the world is referencing today. As it turns out, the old food pyramid was wrong, and it's been changed.

Back in the day, the lower level of the food pyramid was designated to grains which is now the home of fruits and veggies. In fact, nutrition-ists suggest having 8 or 9 servings of fruit and vegetables per day. One or two of these servings can be fruit, and the rest should be cruciferous vegetables. These include celery, cucumber, kale, cauliflower, cabbage, Brussel sprouts, and broccoli, for starters.

It's also recommended to restrict dairy and grains in your diet. Why? What most people don't like to talk about is the effect dairy has on the body. It can irritate joint tissue and cause stomach upset in older people. Grains do not have to be completely left out but keep grain consumption to whole grains when you eat them. Consider whole oats, barley, wheat, quinoa, brown rice, and rye. If you love white rice, then reduce your consumption by making cauliflower rice and mixing it into your white rice for more volume. Avoid red meat. Unfortunately, red meat is one of the culprits of inflammation in the body. This is because of the high saturated fat content in red meats.

Control Your Weight

You were born with a skeleton to support you, and it's your responsibility to ensure that you don't overload that skeleton. Being overweight doesn't mean that your supportive frame will simply grow to keep up. All you're doing is placing unnecessary weight on your muscles and joints. This can present itself in poor maneuverability and pain in the knees, back, and feet.

For every pound of weight you lose, you relieve your body of four pounds of pressure. Stretching is the first step towards getting more active so you can shed a few extra pounds. Most people think that stretching doesn't lead to weight loss, but we beg to differ. Here's a realistic look at how many calories you can expect to burn with daily stretching.

- A 125-pound person can burn 70 calories doing a 30-minute stretching regime.
- A 150-pound person can burn 34 calories doing a 30-minute seated stretching program and 85 calories doing a standing stretching workout.

Not too bad, right?

POSTURE AND HOW IT AFFECTS YOUR BODY

If your mother or teacher ever hissed at you, "stand up straight!" it was pretty good advice. Slouching is something most people do over a lifetime. Sitting and standing up straight is essential for a healthy spine, but it's also good for eliminating muscular aches and pains in the neck, back, and arms. When the muscles are out of alignment, thanks to poor posture, all the muscles work harder than they have to, leading to strains, fatigue, and aches. (chances are that you just corrected your posture by reading this).

If you have never paid much attention to your posture, it can be hard to suddenly make changes, and let's be honest, after years of slouching or hunching, your muscles aren't nearly as strong as they should be. Stretching makes it easier to correct your posture by strengthening the muscles required to hold you up straight and keep your spine and muscles in alignment. If you have poor posture which doesn't look attractive and is causing aches and pains, stretching is the first step you should take to rectify it. Saloni Doshi, a physical therapist at the Harvard-affiliated Brigham and Women's Hospital, says, "Better posture is often just a matter of changing your activities and strengthening your muscles," and we couldn't agree more. You can read more on Saloni Doshi's perspective here: https://tinyurl.com/43nkxdje

Slow, consistent stretches are best to do when working on posture. Getting your back and legs used to extending to their total reach will help you the most.

Injuries

People in their 50s face the constant fear of injury. Is catching your granddaughter as she leaps into your arms going to pull a muscle in your back? Will you slip down the slanting path because you're just not strong enough to be sturdy on your feet anymore?

Injuries are a fact of life, but you don't have to be the most common victim of them. With regular stretching, your muscles become stronger, more flexible, and primed for sudden action or heavy lifting. Stretching exercises that prevent injury are all the stretches that prime the main muscle groups before you work them. If you want to enhance your balance skills, various stretching exercises that strengthen the core can help with that.

Below are two of our favorite anti-injury stretches:

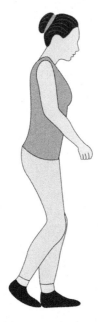

Figure 4-1 HEEL-TOE WALKING

1. Heel to Toe Walking

This is a great stretching exercise for improved balance.

- Position your right foot straight in front of your left foot so that your heel touches the top of your left foot.
- Move your left foot in front of your right foot while pushing

your weight firmly into your heel. Feel your weight create a stretch.
- Now, push all your weight onto your toes.
- Then, repeat this with the other foot.
- Do twenty steps like this.

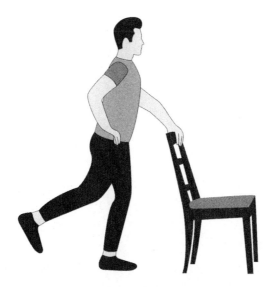

Figure 4-2 BACK LEG RAISES

2. Back Leg Raises

This stretch strengthens the lower back, making it less prone to injuries.

- Stand up straight behind a chair.
- With a slow movement, lift your left leg straight back without bending your knees or pointing your toes.
- Keep your leg straight back for three seconds and then return to the start position.
- Repeat this stretch ten times and then switch to the right leg.

Body Alignment

Body alignment is how the head, shoulders, spine, hips, knees, and ankles relate and line up. When the body is properly aligned, your spine is relieved of extra stress, improving posture while alleviating muscular and joint-related aches and pains. Poor body alignment can lead to the following:

- Chronic back, neck, and shoulder pain
- Carpal tunnel syndrome
- Sciatica
- stiffness
- Headaches
- Fatigue
- Muscle atrophy and weakness
- Difficulty breathing
- Foot, knee, hip, and back injuries
- Irritable bowel syndrome
- Impingement and nerve compression
- Falling

If you're not in alignment, there are stretches you can do to get into better alignment. In addition, there are tests you can do at home to see if you are appropriately aligned.

How to check your body alignment at home:

1. Walk around your home while noticing how your feet are positioned.

The progressive angle of your foot should create a 4 to 7-degree angle. There should be a centerline from your heel to the second toe from your big toe. To notice this, you will have to examine yourself carefully.

Check to see if the toes on one side of your body are pointed out more than on the other side of your body. Then check to see if both sides are pointed out more than a 7-degree angle. If they are, then you might be out of alignment in your lower body. You may be using different muscles than you should be for specific movements, making you more prone to injuries and pain in your ankles, feet, knees, hips, and lower back.

2. Check your frontal posture.

To do this, simply look at yourself in the mirror. There are a few things you're looking for. First, check that both of your shoulders are level with each other. If one shoulder is higher than the other, you might have an alignment problem caused by a muscular imbalance.

Another area to check while looking in the mirror is to see if your nose lines up with your belly button. If this is angled, then that is an indicator your spine might not be appropriately aligned. A poorly aligned spine is prone to injury.

3. Turn your body sideways and look in the mirror.

Now, you're looking at your lateral posture. Check to make sure the opening of your ear is in line with the bump at the top edge of your shoulder joint. Your shoulder joint should line up with the boney bump of your hip. If these three points are not in line, your alignment is out. Physical therapists often advise specific stretches to rectify this problem.

4. Check your pelvis.

To check your pelvis, find the two boney bumps located on the front and back of either side of your pelvis. If these are positioned in a horizontal line in the mirror, then your pelvis is aligned.

Certain stretches can help you with overall body alignment. Below we give you a sneak peek by presenting you with two to try out at home.

Chin Tucks & Juts

You can do this stretch while you are sitting or standing. It aligns the bones in the spinal area, starting with the neck.

Sit down on a sturdy chair or stand up straight. Pull your chin backward as if trying to create a double-chin face. Now, gently push your chin forward in the opposite direction. Repeat this movement six to eight times.

Spinal Extensions

This stretch is good for spinal alignment. Sit on a chair with your arms at your sides and your spine in a neutral position. Breathe in deeply while you sit up and straighten your back. Breathe out as you relax and let your spine return to a neutral position. Repeat this exercise ten times.

Now that you're all clued up on how stretching can help get your posture into alignment and rid your body of aches and pains, let's move on to chapter four: *Types of Stretching.*

4

TYPES OF STRETCHING

Wouldn't it be nice if all you had to do was wipe the sleep out of your eyes, enjoy a long stretch in the morning, and your entire body would be primed and ready for the day? That would be living the dream, even for people still in the paddling pool of aging (those kids in their 30s, you know!).

 We do different stretches throughout our lifespans.

First, there are morning stretches, usually accompanied by a yawn and (hopefully) the smell of a fresh pot of coffee.

Then there are stretches you do every couple of hours over the workday to keep your muscles mobile and flexible (accompanied by moans and groans of all the work piling up). And then there are the stretches you do before exercise, after exercise, and as exercise. All of these stretches that are very much part of our everyday lives can divide into two main groups: Static stretching (this is done without moving, think of stretching and holding), and Dynamic stretching (this is done with movement, think of fluid and repetitive stretching motions).

In your quest for a stronger, healthier, and more flexible you, we encourage you to indulge in both dynamic and static stretching. There's no official requirement for you to know the precise intricacies of both stretch types – there certainly won't be a test at the end of this book, but you should understand what is happening when you do these stretches and why they are important; for your 50+ body. When you carry out a static stretch, which is done in one position and with the muscle held for a certain amount of seconds before it's relaxed, you're extending the muscle. If there were a test, we would give three gold stars to whoever could tell us *why* this stretch is important for a 50+er.

STATIC STRETCHING

Static stretching elongates and extends the muscle. For a 50+ club member, that means improved flexibility and a greater range of motion. It also means stress and tension relief from your muscles so that your body can be more relaxed and your muscles and joints can fall into better alignment.

Sometimes it can seem like you need a medical or physiotherapy qualification to understand just what's happening when you carry out a type of stretch. But you don't! To make the science behind static stretching easier to understand, we've broken down the sub-stretches that fall into this category below.

Traditional

This is a slow and steady stretch where a group of muscles is put under tension, held in place, then slowly relaxed. Then the body is moved once more to increase tension on the muscles and held in position to allow for the muscles to elongate. The aim is to hold the muscle stretched between fifteen and twenty seconds. This is a great form of stretching for 50+ers because it's slow and steady, easy to do, and there's minimal risk of injury.

Assisted Static Stretching

This is also referred to as passive stretching. In such instances, you would have the help of another person or equipment to intensify the stretch. This movement will stretch the muscle slightly further than if you just did a static stretch unaided. As a result, there is a risk of injury if the muscle is pushed too far.

Active Stretching

This type of stretching uses the power of the opposing muscles to stretch a certain muscle or group of muscles. The stretched muscles are relaxed by the contraction of the opposing muscles. You can try an active stretch at home as follows:

- Stand in one position and make sure that you're well balanced.
- Raise one leg in front of you as high as you can.
- Maintain this position without holding onto anything or getting assistance from anyone. Use the strength of the opposing muscles to hold you in position.
- After holding this position for fifteen seconds, lower your leg down to the original position.

Proprioceptive Neuromuscular Facilitation, aka PNF

You can thank a certain Dr. Herman Kabat for this one. He developed the stretch for polio patients in the 1940s to help them develop more flexibility and mobility. This stretch is a little more intense than the others as you push your muscle to its limit but stop before you injure yourself or strain the muscle. There should be a fifteen-second rest between each of these stretches, which must be held for 30 seconds at a time.

Isometric Static Stretching

While isometric stretching is similar to PNF, it is actually more intense and requires more strength. Because of this, it is only recommended for people who know what they are doing and who are already fully developed (not for children). With isometric stretching, each muscle group is stretched and held for around fifteen seconds. There is a twenty-second rest between stretches. These stretches are very demanding on your muscles. Using a resistance band is a form of isometric stretching.

Advice for Static Stretching

- Warm up your muscles before stretching.
- Stretch all areas slowly and gently.
- Make sure you are well-balanced before you start.
- Don't aim for pain. Pain is not a sign of a good stretch.
- Focus on the muscle you're stretching.
- Pay attention to your posture while stretching.

DYNAMIC STRETCHING

Dynamic stretching is a little different in that it requires fluid movements. Essentially, you're measuring how far you can turn, reach or bend when you're doing dynamic stretches. Your aim is to achieve maximum range of motion and flexibility. At first, you might try five stretches and try to work your way up to ten. If you're just getting active again, start with a few and aim to keep adding to your stretches as the days go by. If you're going to play a sport such as soccer, basketball, tennis, or even go for a run, dynamic stretching can be beneficial. It prepares the muscle for several repetitions of a movement.

Types of Dynamic Stretches

Unlike static stretching, which improves flexibility and range of motion, dynamic stretching improves speed, acceleration, and agility. It gives the muscle the power to change directions quickly and even come to a halt on command. The muscle is ready for whatever it encounters. These types of dynamic stretches include:

Ballistic stretching is not a common form of stretching because of the high risk of injury often associated with it. It involves bouncing motions, which have no place in your stretch routine, as we have already told you. We don't recommend trying this type of stretching at home.

Active Isolated Stretches AI was developed by Al Mattes and is a relatively new form of stretching. This stretch works for the most part by well-trained or professional athletes and is only held for a few seconds. This works by forcing the stretched muscles to relax by contracting the opposing muscles, thus releasing tight muscles.

Resistance stretching is a form of stretching that contracts and extends the muscle at the same time. These stretches work through an entire muscle group and extend the range of motion during the contraction, thus strengthening the muscle. Someone with sore shoulders could do a dynamic shoulder stretch to relax the muscles and reduce pain. This is how you do it.

- Relax both of your shoulders while standing with your feet shoulder-width apart.
- Position one arm across your body and hold it in place with your other arm, just above your elbow.
- Pull your arm gently towards your body and notice the slight stretch in the back of the shoulder. Repeat this stretch a few times on both sides for the best results.

HOW DO WE BREATHE AND STRETCH?

If someone asked you how you breathe when you stretch, you'd probably wonder what they meant. How do you breathe? What an absurd question! The same way you normally do, right? Unfortunately, that's where you're wrong. Most people find that they hold their breath when they do an exercise, whether it is a weighted exercise or a simple stretch. And we're willing to bet you're the same. If you've ever experienced pain, upset, panic, or anger in your life, someone might have said to you, "Just breathe through it!" And that's because breathing is at the very heart of everything we do. If you've got your breathing under control, you're in control. And this is how you need to be when you're stretching. Relaxed but in control.

While it might seem like an unimportant aspect of stretching and exercising, breathing is actually essential to the process. If you're not breathing correctly, you're not getting the most out of the exercise – what's the point of that?! Breathing delivers oxygen to the rest of your body, ensuring that your muscles and organs are operating at peak potential when you're putting them to work. Deep breaths also tell the body you are calm and relaxed, which also means you're less likely to suffer an injury from being rigid, stiff, or tense. The rule of thumb is to exhale on exertion. This means that you should breathe out when you're working the hardest. When stretching, exhale as you deepen into the stretch you are doing.

IF YOU ARE NEW TO STRETCHING

If you're new to the art of stretching, don't let your lack of know-how and experience scare you off. Everyone was new to it at some point, so you are not alone at all. Many people have been there before you, and believe it not; many people will be new to stretching after you! The most significant piece of advice we can give you is to be gentle without mistaking your 50+ body for an overly delicate piece of equipment. Just because you're 50+, it doesn't mean you're fragile; it just means you have to take care to do the stretches and exercises the right way. You will be surprised what your body can achieve if you adopt a can-do mindset and just do it. Here's what all newbies to stretching should keep in mind:

Don't try to be a hero. We know you want to run into the room, slide down onto your knees, and bound right back up again like you're Tom Cruise in *Risky Business*, but that's only going to end in pain and disappointment for you. Maybe that's something to work your way up to and not try on the first stretch day. Easy does it because the slower you go and the more you practice, the easier it will be and the more flexible you will become.

Stop comparing your flexibility to other people. If you look across the workout room and see another 50+er putting their leg behind their head and achieving all manner of outstanding pretzel-like shapes with their body, this isn't a sign that you have to be the same. How far you stretch and how flexible you are is relative to your life. Do you really need to stretch your leg behind your head? It would be a great trick to show the grandkids, but they would probably prefer a grandmother or grandfather who can pick them up, push them on the swing or have a jog around the garden with them.

Never rock or bounce while stretching. It might feel like you are working your muscle more intensely when all you're really doing is welcoming an injury. Rocking and bouncing can push beyond the range of motion which can be detrimental. Be consistent. Stretching once a week is just not enough. At the very least, you should practice your full stretch routine three times a week, but we recommend doing at least some stretching every single day.

GETTING STARTED

And here, ladies and gents, is where the real work begins. Now that you're equipped with the many reasons why you should be doing stretching, you're on the precipice of taking the first step and actually getting started. Now is the time to bid a fond farewell to all the excuses of the past. Today is the day you say bye-bye to the aches, pains, and negative thought patterns that you meekly accepted as part of life on your 50th birthday. You're not a statistic. You're not "old." Old is a state of mind, and we're about to teach you how to train your body through simple daily stretches that will leave you slimmer, trimmer, stronger, and more energetic than you've been in years.

First things first, you need to prepare for stretching, plan a stretching routine, and understand what healthy aging is all about – all of which is covered in Chapter five.

Then, and only then, can we move onto Chapter six that covers strategic stretching that also happens to aid you in the top ten activities people in the 50+ club just happen to enjoy!

Let's page over to Chapter five: *Active Living for the 50+ Club.*

5

ACTIVE LIVING FOR THE 50+ CLUB

You get to choose your quality of life right now – this is a sentiment that we hold close to our hearts. If we repeated (or even if we chanted) this 100 times or more, it would not be enough. These words ring true at any age, but they really start hitting home when you reach your 50s. Once you cross over the invisible border into 50-land, you step into one of the largest demographics in the world. And yet, no two bodies are the same in this demographic.

A recent AARP (American Association of Retired Persons) study tells us much of the following…

Americans over 50 are responsible for massive contributions to the economy. We're talking about an over $8 trillion economic contribution in 2020 alone! This statistic puts our little 50+ club just behind the United States and China when measured by GDP. And this economic impact is sure to grow significantly in years to come. It is predicted that we will be contributing more than $28 trillion to the economy by 2050 as Generation Z and millennials reach 50 in the 2030s and the late 2040s.

Another interesting statistic reported is that people over the age of 50 were also responsible for $745 billion worth of unpaid activities in 2018 in ways that benefit society and the world around them. By unpaid activities, we're referring to all the services we provide without charging a cent!

Specifically, we provide caregiving for loved ones, continue to help raise grandchildren, and volunteer countless hours of our time for various causes and events. People in our age bracket spark new ideas, have purchasing power, and contribute services across the world economy. We contribute to the nation's economy that we reside in, regardless of where we live, and many of us are active in local government. Often after retirement, some over 50 keep working and contributing to their next career.

You are not in this newfound age group by yourself. We are a force to reckon with, and for you to be at the top of your game, we have written this book to help you get into the best shape of your life so you can join the rest of us who are fighting fit!

It all begins with stretching.

You have the choice right here, right now, to choose to live a whole life for possibly the next 50 years. Picture that. You actually may have another 50 years to live in a healthy, strong, and vibrant way. If you could choose to be healthy and robust for the next 50 years, you would prefer that path. Scratch that – you would absolutely adore that path. These choices are in your control. Right here, right now!

NO TWO BODIES ARE THE SAME

Just like a snowflake, each individual is different. Science cannot fully explain why one person gets one result from stretching or a specific diet, and another person doing the same thing will get a completely different outcome. Our bodies are different in how they react and process activities, food, and information. When it comes to stretching, consistency is the key. If you become discouraged along the way, remember to stretch every day, no matter what other activities you do. The best advice when working out or stretching is not to compare yourself with others. This concept may be difficult when working with a group or comparing notes, but it is sound advice.

It's like playing golf. Unless you are a professional golfer, you are playing golf to beat your last score. You are competing against your-self. Stretching is much the same as a round of golf. You are extending your stretch just a little further or holding a problematic movement for just a few seconds longer. Remember to never over-extend your muscles. A stretching routine is critical for anyone 50+ because it keeps your muscles flexible and can thoroughly perform their range of motion. The entire range of motion is vital to be able to complete the activity you wish to do. Stretching can make that happen when you do *your* personal best. Some people in the 50+ group love to stretch, and then some people dislike it very much - for different reasons. It could be old habits of negative coaching, a little adult ADHD, boredom, or the act of stretching is keeping you from getting to the good stuff of the activity, etc.

Whatever the case, it is essential right now to figure out a way to love stretching. Think of stretching as a lifeline to your future. Stretching is the key to not falling at age 80 or 90. Stretching will make sure you can dance at your grandson's wedding! Picture dancing at age 75 or 80 when you are stretching – it's all the motivation you'll need. Even though we all have different bodies, we can benefit from stretching if we do the movement every day. Stretching does not take long, and you do not have to leave your home. If it is -20F outside, you can still stretch and keep your muscles warm. All you really need is to make a stretching routine that you can do anywhere, and we will help you with that in Chapter 6.

YOUR FITNESS JOURNEY

Starting a fitness journey is the best gift you can give yourself. Phys-ical activity beginning with a quality stretching program can reduce your risk of getting chronic diseases, improve your balance, your coordination, and help you lose weight. You will notice improvements in sleeping habits and increased energy levels almost immediately. By immediately, we mean within the span of one or two weeks. The first thing you should do to start your fitness journey is to assess exactly where you are right now. Record some baseline scores for yourself. As far as stretching goes, record your measurements on your extensions (how far you can stretch). How far can you extend each of your leg and arm muscles during stretches? Take your measurements.

Weight control isn't always about losing weight. Muscle weighs more than fat. What matters is how you feel and what your body can do. Here is a list for an example of suggested measurements you can take:

- Your heart rate before and straight after walking briskly for 1 mile (1.6 kilometers)
- How many minutes it takes you to walk 1 mile, or how long it takes you to run 1.5 miles (2.41 kilometers)
- How many pushups you can do at one time (standard or modified)
- How far you can stretch forward if you're sitting on the ground with your legs straight
- Your waist
- Your BMI (this is your body mass index)
- Your resting heart rate

Design Your Daily Stretching Program

Your stretching should happen before your daily fitness routine. Stretching will significantly impact your fitness level, flexibility, and overall body mobility if done daily. As a 50+er, doing anything you can to increase mobility is a must! Mobility increases your chances for continued fitness and independence throughout life. We are passionate about this because stretching vs. less movement is directly related to more knee and hip injuries down the road for our older citizens. Some people never recover after a fall past 70 if they are not in good physical condition. This should be reason enough to put this book down and start stretching immediately! But you can't because you don't have a plan or program, which brings us to the next bit – how to plan.

 When you plan your stretching program, consider your goals. What are your goals now that you have joined the 50+ club?

Are you trying to lose weight? Do you want to be healthier so you can do more with your kids and grandkids? What about bucket list items? Perhaps there is a long hike or bike ride on your list, or maybe there's a destination you've always wished to visit, but there will be a lot of walking or cycling involved. People frequently have an extensive tour they wish to do after retirement, and then they discover by the time they retire, they are not up to the rigors of a long trip.

When you think about goals, also consider your lifetime independence. You don't want to be a person who is overly concerned about doing extracurricular activities because you are afraid of falling. Having goals helps you to stay motivated and will also help you to gauge your progress. When designing your stretching and fitness program, it should include a balanced routine. If you are a healthy adult, you should have at least 150 minutes of moderate aerobic activity weekly. If you don't have time for 150 minutes, you can do 75 minutes of vigorous exercise weekly. We want to add that you should also have at least 20 minutes for stretching each day.

If stretching becomes a part of your daily fitness routine, you will see even more significant health benefits. We cannot stress enough how much stretching will help you stay on your feet and keep moving forward doing the things you love to do! If you are just beginning to exercise, you are not alone. Many people in our club are just now finding the time to become active again. Even small amounts of physical activity are helpful. If you can't hit those target amounts of 150 minutes at first, do not sweat the small stuff! Any minutes you can do any physical activity are better than none, and if you're doing more than you managed to do yesterday, last week, or even last month – that's progress! Be proud that you are getting back into action. Your journey of health and activity is a marathon, not a sprint!

Try to schedule activities into your day even if you are busy. Walk up the steps instead of opting to take an elevator. Park further away in a parking lot from the door. Walk your dog more often – it will be good for both of you. Find a way to make stretching and exercise a personal challenge. While you are stretching, see if you can reach just slightly further than the day before. When starting a lifetime stretching and fitness program, you should choose activities you enjoy. The more you enjoy your activities, the more you will want to be actively engaged in movement.

Midlife is Revolutionized by Stretching

The above heading is a statement that we do not make lightly. We base our reputations on it. Your life can be revolutionized by stretching, and you will reap more benefits than we could ever put into one book. However, we are going to list eight life-changing benefits we get from stretching. Take them to heart because soon they will be *your* benefits, too!

Stretching improves flexibility.

We have talked about flexibility over and over, but perhaps we haven't discussed how improving flexibility is life-changing after 50. You may think you want to take it easier at this age, but don't fall into that mindset. Taking it easy and watching too much TV in your 50s is what will possibly earn you a broken hip with an innocent wrong step at age 80.

Activity is the key to health, and stretching is critical to being able to stay active. Exercise physiologist, John Ford, owner of JFK Fitness and Health in New York City, has stated, "Stretching can help increase your range of motion—both temporarily and in the long term." Here is the kicker. It does not work stretching one day and expecting it to last. The gains of stretching will not last unless they are repeated *every day*. To lengthen your muscles and keep your range of motion long term, you have to stretch every day for six days each week. This is essential if you want to see a change and meet your goals.

Stretching can help your muscles work when you are doing things you enjoy.

If you stick with a stretching routine, you will also see a greater rate in your performance when you do all your favorite things. If you love to play golf, we will almost bet your golf rounds are going to improve. You might notice your serve in pickleball is more brutal, and your charge to the net is a little bit faster.

We are talking about competitive sports in midlife (imagine that!), and you are more competitive because your muscles are more stretched out. They are ready to go when they are called on to do their job. You will notice that when you increase your flexibility and your muscles have more power, you have the opportunity to be more competitive, no matter what your age.

Stretching makes everyday life easier.

Whether it's working in the garden or on the job, you will have more energy thanks to stretching. Because of your stretching routine, your extended muscles and greater flexibility will make everyday tasks notably easier. Imagine effortlessly standing up from your weeding kneepad while doing a spot of gardening to warmly welcome your daughter and grandkids in!

Some people by age 70 even have a difficult time getting in and out of the car. You don't want to be in the category. Leaning, bending, squatting are all motions we still need to do as we age in our day-to-day life.

Choose to stay mobile and flexible using stretching and extending your muscles, which ultimately boosts flexibility. These actions are life-changing. If you saw a stiff person struggling with mobility and asked them if they would have stretched 20 years previously if they knew it would solve their flexibility and mobility issues, what do you think their answer would be? They'd probably be looking for a time machine!

Stretching gets you ready for a workout.

If you are getting ready for a dynamic workout (workouts that require movement), dynamic stretches will help you achieve more during this workout. Like we discussed in Chapter 4, dynamic stretches will help your body prepare for moving faster during an activity or a sport.

These stretches help you gradually move from slow to fast. The gradual movement allows your body to work more efficiently to absorb higher impact. You may experience impacts during workouts or sporting competitions. Dynamic stretches also fire up your brain! There is a mind-muscle connection, and research shows people who do dynamic stretching when they enter their 50s and beyond keep their memory and body sharp well into their 80s and 90s. This bodes well for you! It's never too late to get started!

Stretching will increase your stability and decrease your risk of falling.

If we sound like we are beating the same drum, we are because it is essential. How many older people lose their independence because of falls? We'll answer that for you – many!

 Stretching will increase your range of motion. If you are short in your range of motion, it increases the likelihood of falling and becoming injured.

With a daily stretching program, coordination and reflexes also improve. Stretching helps to let you know what imbalances you need to deal with to stabilize your body. If you notice one leg or one hip lunges better than the other, you can concentrate on stretching the stiffer side that's less able to move. This movement will, in turn, stabilize the weaker side of your body. Be mindful of how your body feels when you stretch, and you will gain more knowledge about how your body will perform. Pay attention to your strong and weak sides and give those weak sides a little extra attention.

Stretching also decreases the rate of injuries while you are doing the activities you love to do. Randi Blackmon, ACSM-certified exercise physiologist in Houston, Texas, stated, "To compensate for a shortened range of motion, you might lean forward, which could cause you to stress your back, or turn your knees in, which could cause pain in those joints on the outside." Moving and doing activities pain-free is worth the stretch daily and before you go into a full-on workout. You can read more on this here: https://www.self.com/story/benefits-of-stretching

Stretching calms your body after exercise.

It is critical to give your body time to calm down after exercise. When you stretch after strenuous activity, you help your body in several ways. First, stretching lowers your heart rate, calms your breathing, and helps lower your adrenaline levels, too. During your cool-down stretching, your body and heart rate calms down to a natural state. We recommend stretching before and after exercise. When using stretching to cool down, remember to breathe deeply. This increases blood flow and delivers nutrients to your body and muscles.

Stretching helps you relax.

Relaxing is one of the mental benefits of stretching. If you give stretching a chance, it will leave you feeling good physically and mentally. Mindful stretching is essential to your mental well-being. This activity can reduce chronic stress – which means it's a pretty good replacement for chocolate! We all know that good chocolate is hard to beat but stretching is a Zen activity that will bring you to a calm state of being without putting on weight – so you tell us which is better? Stretching or chocolate?

If you pair your stretching with deep breathing, it can be meditational. Mentally let go of the things that stress you each time you breathe out. Do each stretch intentionally, trying to extend your muscles a little further without causing pain or injury. When you stretch in an intentional, mindful way, it can give you the mental boost you needed to tackle the challenges of 50+ life.

Stretching is an act of self-care.

Self-care has become quite a buzzword in recent years and it becomes even more of a buzzword when you reach 50+. You need self-care in your 50's more than any other time of your life!

If you are just entering your 50s, it is quite possible you could live another 50 years and of course, you want to live those extra 50 years well! Extended healthy living is a legacy of hope you can pass on to your children and grandchildren. By your example, they too can live a healthy, active, and long life. Stretching is a gift you give to yourself and your loved ones too. The longer you can take care of yourself, the longer you can enjoy your life and continue to contribute to the world.

BUILDING A POSITIVE MENTAL ATTITUDE (PMA)

As 50+ers ourselves, we have been in a unique position to observe others in our club. We have noticed that people tend to split into two distinct groups when they enter their golden years.

In group one, the members seem to enjoy activities and new ideas about eating and nutrition. In group two, the members tend to sway more toward being less active.

We did discuss this in earlier chapters and if this sounds judgmental, bear with us for a moment because it also has a great deal to do with a person's mental attitude. As you age, you begin making choices or directions to travel along in life. You choose who to have as friends, your jobs, how to raise children, and where to live. You make many decisions daily that affect your outcomes later in life.

Life just doesn't happen to you. You make choices. You recognize illness or accidents occur. But you choose how you recover eventually. At first, a horrible loss may knock you completely down, but you decide whether to get back up in a fresh new way or to be bitter about the experience called life. The people who keep choosing to try new things and who continue to reinvent themselves as they age are the ones who tend to gravitate toward others who are doing the same things. These are the 50+ individuals who have a positive mental attitude (PMA).

PMA will is one of the critical factors of having a long, happy life. Happy people tend to want to be around other happy people. It's not that they ignore the needs of the world; quite the opposite. These people are usually very active in their communities and worldwide for various causes because of their eternal optimism about the possibility of the future. There are concrete benefits to having a positive mental attitude. They are:

- Longer life
- Better psychological and physical health
- Fewer colds
- Lower rates of depression
- Higher energy levels
- Better stress management and coping skills
- Better quality of life
- Quicker recovery from injury or illness

If you want to develop a positive mental attitude, or if your PMA needs a little tweaking, there are some actions you can take today to gain some positivity in your life. You are not too old or too young to change - that's a promise!

Focus on the good things.

Difficulties are quite simply a part of life - everyone has them. We are all faced with difficulty. Focus on what you can control and deal with that. Try to find something positive to think about each day. If something doesn't go well, focus on what *does* go well.

Practice gratitude.

We have never met anyone who kept a gratitude journal who did not have a positive mental attitude. Start with writing down just three things you are thankful for each day. Think of people, moments, or something that brings you comfort. Items can be as simple as a glass of water or the bird that flew by your window.

Try see the funny side of life and situations.

It is a fact that people who laugh have lower stress levels. Try to find humor even when things may not be funny. Some friends told us that when they were burying a beloved uncle, they could overhear two of the sisters, their aunts, getting into a spat on the way to the gravesite. His wife, their other sister, had no idea. For some reason, it struck them funny. They have not quit laughing about it to this day.

Spend time with positive people.

Both negativity and positivity are contagious. Which one do you want to catch? You become like the people you choose to spend time with even in adulthood. Make good choices to enjoy a longer life.

Talk nicely to yourself.

It would help if you were your own biggest cheerleader. You spend the most time with yourself, so if the voice in your head is negative, it will have a negative impact on how you think and feel. Research shows that even a tiny shift in how you talk to yourself will help boost your attitude and the way you behave under stress. Don't say or think things about yourself that you wouldn't say to or about someone else.

Identify your areas of negativity.

Be honest with yourself about your negative behaviors. Don't use this as a self-bashing session, but rather as a way of recognizing when you're negative and should adjust your approach.

Begin every day on a positive note.

Start your morning differently - start it by doing something that leaves you feeling good. Of course, a morning, meditative stretch is always a great idea! Do something to start the day that leaves you feeling good about who you are.

Negative thinking has many side effects, such as headaches, colon problems, stomach aches, fatigue, difficulty sleeping, and body aches. Stress, anger, and holding in hostility can lead to heart disease, heart attack, dementia, and stroke. If you are consumed with negative thinking, it's time to take steps towards adopting a more positive approach to daily life.

On the other hand, a positive mental attitude will go a long way toward increasing your health and longevity. This life is your life, and if you want to enjoy a healthy and happy life and get a leg up toward achieving your fitness and health goals, it's time to start thinking more positively!

Quality of Life

The cornerstone of the 50+ club is our desire to enjoy an exceptional quality of life. The big take-home concept is that you are deciding what your quality of life is now and what it will be in the future. This is power. The question we present to you: How are you going to use this power?

First things first, good food equals good quality of life. It is your responsibility now to eat the best food you can to power your body. Good nutrition will ensure that your machine works at its best. Your body should be eating a diet of mainly vegetables and fruit to work at its highest capacity. Use the food pyramid to complete your daily requirements each day and ensure that you consume 6 to 8 glasses of water, too.

In addition to healthy eating, you also need to make sure that you don't stop moving. Stretching, which is ideal for boosting flexibility must be done daily to ensure that you can participate in activities and maintain your independence well into your 60s, 70s, and beyond. Stretching will also ensure you experience fewer injuries and have more fun with the people you love. Your quality of life is up to you.

Full Engagement

If you are stretching, doing activities, and eating healthy each day, you will find that your body experiences full engagement. By full engagement, we refer to your body functioning at peak performance while you are also mentally and physically engaged in your life. You're actually living – not just existing.

The 50+ club steals the show when we take over the tennis courts, the bike trails, and the gyms. Research shows that the 50+ demographic is becoming one of the largest consumers of activewear and accessories, and that's not because gym wear is comfy to wear around the house! It's because we're becoming fully engaged, separately and together. We're working out, we're getting fit, and we're living life 50+!

Healthy Aging

Almost everything in research that points to healthy aging refers to physical activity as a significant contributing factor. The truth is that some people do not enjoy doing lots of physical activity – we get that - but if you can get yourself on a daily stretching routine and have a healthy, balanced diet, you are most likely to approach aging healthily.

Any physical activity that keeps your body moving will contribute to your health and mental well-being. We cannot stress enough that stretching and flexibility training will keep your body limber and your muscles extended. You will have freedom of movement with less risk of injury as you get older. Evidence now suggests that people who begin exercise training in later life (in their 60s and 70s) can also experience improved heart function.

In the Baltimore Longitudinal Study of Aging, researchers observed a decreased risk of a coronary event, such as a heart attack, if people over 50 took part in higher intensity leisure-time physical activities. These activities include lap swimming, bike riding, or running, and of course, social activities. People tend to age better when they are having fun with others. Spending time with friends, children, and grandchildren seems to round out the 50+ life in a happy, healthy way.

Healthy aging is our goal. The 50+ club is all about enjoying life and aging well at the same time. Having a fitness plan is the way to achieve your fitness goals and live a happy, healthy life, not just in your 50s but well into your 80s and 90s.

With that said, we're about to take the plunge into the real work: the actual stretching—page over to Chapter Six: *Stretches for the Top Ten Activities.*

6

STRETCHES FOR THE TOP TEN ACTIVITIES

A s active 50+ers, we're in a good position to know what others in the 50+ club are up to, now that they have more time on their hands.

We've realized that not all 50+ers are the same. Some like to lace up their running shoes and hit the road as if they're training for a marathon, while others like to do something active, but with a leisure activity focus, like playing golf or doing a bit of gardening.

Gardening | Walking | Jogging | Running | Hiking | Golf | Swimming | Tennis | Pickleball | Cycling

After surveying a large number of our fellow 50+ club members, we compiled a list of the top 10 actives most like to participate in. And then, we designed a program of stretching to help make these activities easier and more enjoyable. We might be getting ahead of ourselves when we say this, but; you're welcome! Hopefully, your favorite activities appear on our list (fingers crossed)!

While some of these could be viewed strictly as exercise, others can be seen as leisure activities and hobbies. What they all have in common, though, is that they involve physical movement.

Unfortunately, another thing they have in common is that they can be activities quickly abandoned by 50+ers who are stiff, in pain, or lack flexibility. If you want to enjoy these activities well into your 60s, 70s, and beyond, stretching is the secret. And our gift to you is a carefully designed routine of stretches for each activity that can help you better enjoy your favorite activities now and for many years to come!

LET'S GET STRETCHING!

In the exercise routines that follow, you will see that some of the same stretches apply to more than one activity. That's because many of the exercises require the same muscle groups and similar movements.

Gardening

GARDENING

There's a lot of bending, hunching, pulling, reaching, pushing, stretching, and carrying when gardening. Your muscles must be warm and ready for a good day's work. For most people in the 50+ club, their garden represents a sanctuary, a place away from the hustle and bustle of everyday life. I know 50+ers who consider gardening to be a little bit of therapy for the soul? Gardening is quite an active sport when you consider the types of activity that go into getting your garden in tip-top shape. You may not even be aware of the muscles used to repot your favorite plant. As you know, strenuous gardening activities such as grass cutting, hedge trimming, and leaf blowing use various muscles in the arms, shoulders, back, and legs. Engaging in these activities without performing the necessary stretches to warm the muscles can lead to muscle strain and unnecessary pain for days after. These stretches are designed to prime your body for a good gardening workout and minimal pain thereafter.

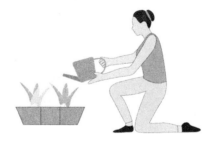

#1 - **Overhead Stretch** - gardening

The overhead stretch works your outer arm muscles. Inhale as you stretch up and exhale when you bring your arms down.

- Reach your arms upward and extend them over your head.
- Keep your palms facing downward.
- Interlock your fingers together.
- Hold the overhead stretch for 10 to 15 seconds.
- Then bring your arms down.
- Repeat this motion 8 to 10 times.

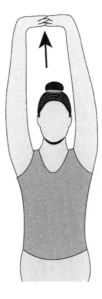

Figure 5-1 OVERHEAD STRETCH

#2 – **Shoulder Raises** - gardening

Shoulder raises are similar to a shrug except slow and intentional. This stretch increases shoulder mobility and brings more flexibility to the back and neck. It targets the trapezius muscles located on either side of your neck and helps with maintaining proper posture and everyday movements like lifting and reaching.

- Keep your arms hanging along the sides of your body.
- Bring your shoulders up slowly, as far as they can go without hurting (this is a dramatic shrug)
- Hold this shrug stance for 10 seconds
- Relax your shoulders.
- Repeat this stretch 6 to 8 times.

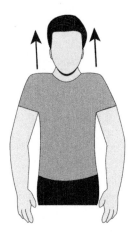

Figure 5-2 SHOULDER RAISES

#3 – Arm Extension Stretch - gardening

This stretch increases flexibility and range of motion.

- Extend your arms in front of you
- Raise your arms to shoulder height
- Turn your palms outward
- Interlock your fingers with the backs of your hands facing you
- Feel the stretch in your arms, shoulders, and upper back
- Hold for a few seconds
- Repeat 6-8 times

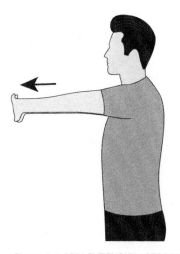

Figure 5-3 ARM EXTENSION STRETCH

#4 – **Tricep Stretch** - gardening

This stretch creates more flexibility in the tricep while increasing mobility in the elbow joint.

- Stand with your feet hip-width apart.
- Bend your knees slightly.
- Raise your left arm in the air and bend your elbow so that your hand drops behind your head.
- Use your right hand to help pull your left elbow.
- Hold this stretch for 10 to 15 seconds
- Repeat the arm stretch with the opposite arm.
- Do at least 6 of these arm stretches on each side.

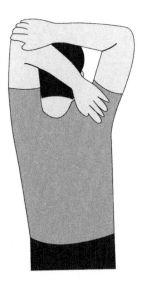

Figure 5-4 TRICEP STRETCH

#5 – **Torso Rotations** - gardening

This stretch relieves lower back-pain, increases flexibility in the back and side muscles, and increases general mobility.

- Stand with your feet shoulder-width apart, and then bend your knees slightly.
- Slowly and <u>gently</u> twist your upper body to the left while looking over your shoulder.
- Do not push too far.
- Hold that twisted stretch for 5 to 10 seconds and then repeat the stretch on the right side.
- Repeat this stretch on the right side.
- You may be tempted to bounce during this exercise, but it's important to focus on a slow, steady, and fluid movement.

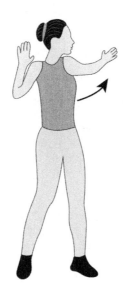

Figure 5-5 TORSO ROTATIONS

#6 – **Standing Side Stretch** - gardening

This stretch relieves tension in muscles, reduces pain, and increases flexibility in the neck and shoulders. Side stretches in the shoulder area also improve mobility.

- Raise your arms above your head.
- Bend your elbows so that each palm now touches the elbow of the opposite arm.
- Tighten your abdominal muscles, and then with a straight back, bend slightly to the left side.
- Feel the muscle stretch on the opposite side and in your shoulders. Hold this stretch for 5 to 10 seconds and then return to the starting position.
- Repeat this stretch on the right-hand side.
- Do at least 8 to 10 stretches on each side.

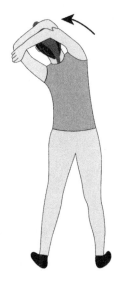

Figure 5-6 STANDING SIDE STRETCH

#7 – **Lower Back Stretch** - gardening

With all the bending, reaching, and pulling involved in gardening, you're in a good position to hurt your lower back. Lower back stretches help to protect you from injury and also ensure greater flexibility in your lower back.

- Stand with your back straight and feet shoulder-width apart.
- Slowly bend torso forward at hips keeping knees slightly bent.
- Relax your arm and neck as you bend.
- Only bend about one-third the way down.
- Feel the slight stretching in the lower back.
- Hold for 10 seconds and return to starting position.
- Repeat this stretch 8 to 10 times.

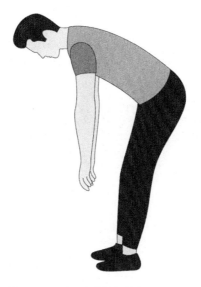

Figure 5-7 LOWER BACK STRETCH

#8 – **Squat Stretch** - gardening

When you bend down to pull out some weeds, pick up your watering can, or get a better vantage point when planting flowers/veggies, you're on your haunches – you're squatting. If you start squatting for long periods on cold muscles that aren't prepared for it, you're going to be stiff and achy the next day. Squat stretches will prepare your muscles for the work and ensure that they enjoy greater flexibility while also strengthening your knees, back, ankles, tendons, and Achilles.

- Stand with your feet shoulder-width apart, angled slightly outwards.
- Squat down as far as you can go without feeling uncomfortable.
- Hold the stretch for 5 seconds and then rise to the starting position.
- Repeat this stretch 8 to 10 times.

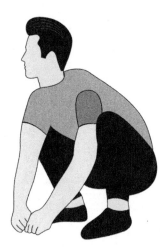

Figure 5-8 SQUAT STRETCH

#9 – **Quad Stretch** - gardening

When gardening, your knees are put to the test. This stretch is essential to develop the muscles around the knee and in the quads while increasing flexibility and mobility.

- Stand in front of a solid object to hold for stability.
- Make sure your feet are shoulder-width apart.
- Place your right hand on the stable object in front.
- Raise right leg up to your buttocks, grab your foot with your left hand.
- Pull your foot up to create a stretch in your quads.
- Hold this stretch for 10 to 15 seconds and then release.
- Switch legs and repeat. Aim to stretch each leg 8 to 10 times.

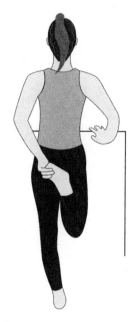

Figure 5-9 QUAD STRETCH

#10 – **Forward Lunge** - gardening

Lunges are a lower body exercise that tone up your body. They help to improve overall fitness that helps to stabilize your muscles and assist with balance and stability.

- Stand upright, look directly ahead with your feet shoulder width apart.
- Your toes should be facing forward.
- Move your right leg forward to take a big step.
- Lower your body until your right thigh is parallel to the floor.
- Press your right heel to drive back up to the upright starting position.
- Repeat the same movement on the left side, then alternate each side 10 times.

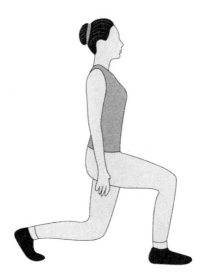

Figure 5-10 FORWARD LUNGE

11 – **Back Arch Stretch** - gardening

This stretch helps to relieve tension in your lower back and loosen up any tightness. At the same time it strengthens your back, hips, chest and shoulders. The aim of this exercise is to promote and improve mobility and increase your flexibility.

- Start positioned on the floor with your hands and knees hip-width apart.
- Arch the back, drawing your belly button up toward your spine while keeping your hands at shoulder-width apart.
- Hold for a brief second.
- Slowly relax the muscles allowing the stomach to naturally fall toward the floor, while exhaling. Keep your shoulders and hips in the very same position.
- Return to the starting position and repeat this motion a total of 10 times.

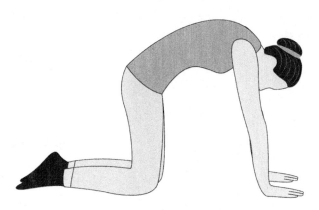

Figure 5-11 BACK ARCH STRETCH

Walk Jog Run

WALK, JOG & RUN

Whether you walk, jog or run, there is nothing better than pulling on your runners and hitting the sidewalk for a feel-good sweat session. Best of all it's an inexpensive activity you can do anywhere, alone or as part of a group. It's a great way to socialize as your feet eat up the miles. However, it also means you are using a range of muscles found in your chest, abdomen, legs, and thighs. All of which work together as you run to keep your body moving forwards. A good warm-up session stretching these muscles will ensure you don't suffer a preventable muscle injury or strain. It also prepares your muscles for the movements they will be doing on repeat for the next few minutes (or however you plan to run, walk, or jog). Before you hit the road or sidewalk, do the following stretches to prepare yourself.

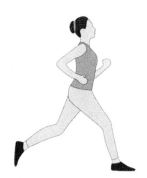

#1 – Chest/Shoulder Stretch - walk, jog, run

This exercise stretches the pectoralis major, deltoids, and biceps muscles. It will improve your back, open up your chest and increase the range of motion of your shoulders. It will also expand your lungs, so you get more oxygen when running or walking.

- Stand with your feet together, relax your arms and breath in.
- With your head upright and shoulders back and down, clasp your hands behind your back.
- Slowly turn your elbows inward as you extend your arms.
- Imagine as if grasping a ball behind you.
- With your chest out and chin in, lift your arms behind you until you feel a stretch.
- Hold for 10 to 15 seconds.

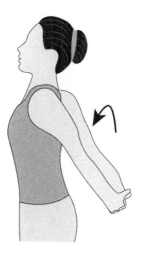

Figure 6-1 CHEST/SHOULDER STRETCH

#2 – **Standing Abdominal Stretch** - walk, jog, run

This exercise stretches your abdominals, latissimus dorsi, obliques, and biceps. It's excellent for loosening up your upper body before a walk or run and is suitable for working on better posture.

- Reach your arms upward extending them overhead.
- Place your palms together.
- Extend your arms upwards and lean back slightly.
- Stay balanced through the stretch.
- Hold the stretch for 10 to 15 seconds.
- Inhale as you stretch up, exhale when lowering arms.
- Repeat 8 to 10 times.

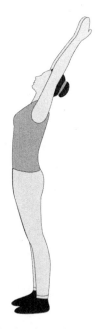

Figure 6-2 STANDING ABDOMINAL STRETCH

#3 – **Torso Twist** - walk, jog, run

This exercise stretches your trunk muscles and improves your core strength, flexibility, stability, and spine mobility. This dynamic movement activates your core and prepares it for motions like walking or running. It's also excellent for reducing low back pain.

- Stand tall with your feet shoulder-width apart, knees slightly bent, and hands placed on your hips.
- Slowly and smoothly rotate the upper body to bring your right shoulder to the front and your left shoulder to the back.
- Hold for a few seconds then slowly and smoothly rotate your upper body in the opposite direction. Bring your left shoulder to the front and your right shoulder to the back.
- Hold for a few seconds and repeat 2 to 3 times.

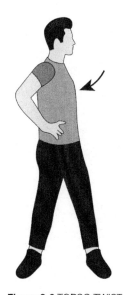

Figure 6-3 TORSO TWIST

#4 – Tricep Stretch - walk, jog, run

This exercise stretches the internal and external obliques, triceps, and latissimus dorsi. It increases your flexibility and helps prevent injuries.

- Stand with feet shoulder-width apart.
- Raise your left arm and bend it at the elbow.
- With elbow pointing upwards drop arm behind your head.
- Grab the left elbow with your right hand and pull to the right.
- Hold this position for 10 to 15 seconds.
- Return to starting position, breath, and repeat on the other side, pulling your right elbow with your left hand.
- Hold again for 10 to 15 seconds.
- Perform 2 to 3 repetitions on each side.

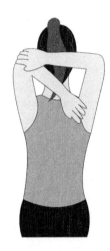

Figure 6-4 TRICEP STRETCH

#5 – Quad Stretch - walk, jog, run

This exercise stretches the quadriceps and anterior tibialis. It helps your quads gain and maintain flexibility and warms up the anterior tibialis to ensure you don't trip over when walking or running.

- Stand on your left foot, grab onto a chair or wall for balance.
- Grasp the top of your right foot with your left hand by bending the right leg up towards your buttocks.
- Pull your foot in towards your right buttock, ensuring your knee is pointing towards the ground.
- Hold this position for 10 to 15 seconds.
- Return to starting position and switch sides.
- Repeat 3 to 4 times on each side.

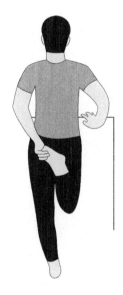

Figure 6-5 QUAD STRETCH

#6 – **Calf Stretch** - walk, jog, run

This exercise stretches your gastrocnemius and soleus muscles which are taxed by walking or running. It will help prevent calf injuries and pain.

- Do this stretch standing in front of a wall while leaning on it with your forearms. Rest your head on your arms.
- Place the right foot in front of you, leg bent.
- Your left leg should be straight out behind you.
- Slowly move your hips forward until you start to feel a stretch in the calf muscle of your left leg.
- Keep the left heel flat and toes pointing straight forward.
- Hold this position for 10 to 15 seconds.
- Switch legs and alternate for 2 repetitions. Ensure you don't bounce or hold your breath.

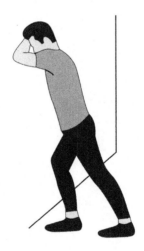

Figure 6-6 CALF STRETCH

#7 – **Hamstring Stretch** - walk, jog, run

This exercise stretches the hamstrings, gluteal, and erector spinae muscles. Warming up these muscles improves your performance and flexibility when walking and running while preventing tightness and pain.

- Stand with your feet hip-width apart and knees slightly bent.
- Bend forward and reach towards your toes.
- Keep your head up and legs straight.
- Hold this position for 10 to 15 seconds.
- Ensure you steadily breathe in and out without holding your breath.

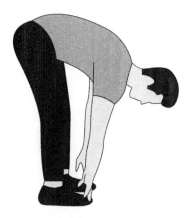

Figure 6-7 HAMSTRING STRETCH

#8 – Hip Flexor Stretch - walk, jog, run

This exercise stretches the hip flexor muscles, which allow flexion on your hip joint. It will improve your mechanics when walking or running and prevent injury and pain on the hips and lower back.

- Start in a standing position. Take a deep step forward using your left foot like you're making an extended lunge.
- Plant your left foot firmly on the ground at a 90-degree angle.
- Your right knee should now be resting gently on the floor.
- Lower your right hip until you feel a stretch without changing position. Place your hands on the floor to avoid overextension or putting too much weight on your hips.
- Hold for 10 to 15 seconds.
- Return to starting position and switch legs.
- Repeat 2 to 3 times on each leg.

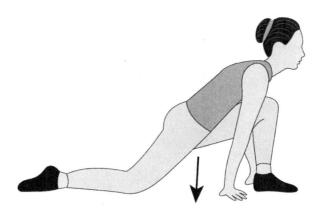

Figure 6-8 HIP FLEXOR STRETCH

#9 – Deep Body-Weight Squat - walk, jog, run

This exercise stretches your hamstrings, glutes, calf muscles, and quadriceps. It's excellent for increasing mobility and strength and improving your functional movement and lower back and pelvic stability.

- Position your feet shoulder-width apart and stand firm.
- Slowly squat down as if you're sitting in a chair.
- Your ankles, knees, and hips should bend in unison while your back remains straight.
- To improve and maintain balance at the lowest depth, use your fingertips to touch the floor in front of you.
- Your feet should remain flat on the ground for the entire movement.
- Hold this position for as long as you can, starting with at least 30 seconds to one minute.

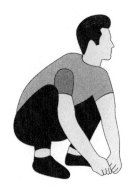

Figure 6-9 DEEP BODY WIEGHT SQUAT

#10 – **Standing Knee to Chest** - walk, jog, run

This stretch is used for your lower back and your hip (lumbar) and improves flexibility. It works on your hamstrings, your inner/outer thighs, and helps to release and tight muscles in those areas.

- Lie down facing the ceiling with both of your legs resting on the floor straight out ahead of you.
- Stand in a straight position (and with body located near a wall or stable object for balance).
- Bring one knee up into your hands and pull toward your chest.
- Hold for a few seconds and lower that same knee back down onto the floor in a resting position.
- Take a breath, then repeat 10 times for each leg.

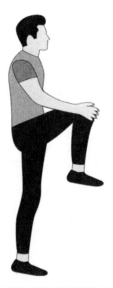

Figure 6-10 STANDING KNEE TO CHEST

Hiking

HIKING

Clambering up over rocks and powering up steep hills or down winding paths presents a few challenges to the 50+ body. Going on a hike, you need your wits about you as who knows what mother nature will throw across your way! The truth is hiking is a great way to get out into the sun while exercising and exploring. But, with all that exploring comes a lot of scrambling over things, ducking under stuff, and maintaining your balance while crossing rough terrain. Balance alone requires good posture and good core strength, all of which is obtained when muscles are properly stretched, warm, and ready to work. Stretching your muscles before a long hike will see you tramping home tired and happy rather than limping home nursing a muscle injury. The following are a few stretches you can do before going on a hike.

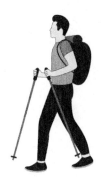

#1 – **Lower Back Stretch** - hiking

Lower back stretches help to protect you from injury and also ensure greater flexibility in your lower back.

- Stand with your back straight and feet approximately shoulder-width apart.
- Slowly bend torso forward at hips and keeping your knees slightly bent.
- Relax your arms and neck as you bend.
- Now bend forward a third of the way and feel slight stretching in your lower back.
- Hold for 10 seconds and return to starting position.
- Repeat this stretch 8 to 10 times.

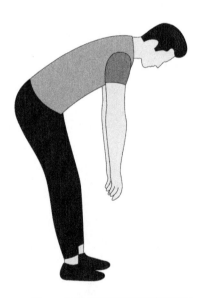

Figure 7-1 LOWER BACK STRETCH

#2 – **Torso Rotations** - hiking

This exercise stretches your trunk muscles and improves your core strength, flexibility, stability, and spine mobility. This dynamic movement activates your core and prepares it for the motions of walking and hiking. It's also excellent for reducing low back pain.

- Stand with your feet shoulder-width apart, and then bend your knees slightly.
- Slowly and <u>gently</u> twist your upper body to the left while looking over your shoulder.
- Do not push too far.
- Hold that twisted stretch for 5 to 10 seconds and then repeat the stretch on the right side.
- Repeat this stretch on the right side.
- You may be tempted to bounce during this exercise, but it's important to focus on a slow, steady and fluid movement.

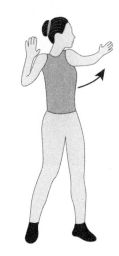

Figure 7-2 TORSO ROTATIONS

#3 – **Hamstring Stretch** - hiking

This stretches the hamstrings, gluteal, and erector spinae muscles to improve your performance and flexibility when hiking while preventing tightness and pain.

- Stand with your feet hip-width apart and knees slightly bent.
- Bend forward and reach towards your toes.
- As you bend forward with fingertips extending to your toes, keep your head in a neutral position.
- Hold this position for 10 to 15 seconds.
- Steadily breathe in and out throughout without holding your breath.

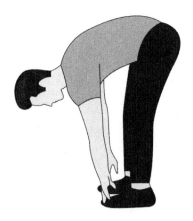

Figure 7-3 HAMSTRING STRETCH

#4 – **Standing Abdominal Stretch** - hiking

This exercise stretches your abdominals, latissimus dorsi, obliques, and biceps. It's excellent for loosening up your upper body before a walk or hike and is suitable for working on better posture as well.

- Reach your arms upward extending them overhead.
- Place your palms together.
- Extend your arms upwards and lean back slightly.
- Stay balanced through the stretch.
- Hold the stretch for 10 to 15 seconds.
- Inhale as you stretch up, exhale when lowering arms.
- Repeat 8 to 10 times.

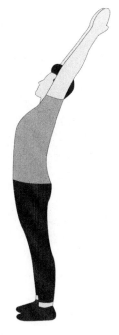

Figure 7-4 STANDING ABDOMINAL STRETCH

#5 – Shoulder Raises - hiking

This exercise stretches the trapezius muscles on either side of your neck. It will stabilize your upper back and neck and improve shoulder movement. Shoulder raises help with maintaining proper posture and everyday movements like lifting and reaching.

- Stand with feet flat on the floor and shoulder-width apart.
- Put your arms on your sides, bend your knees slightly and face straight ahead with chin up and neck straight.
- Slowly bring your shoulders as high up your ears as you can as you inhale.
- Hold for a few seconds.
- Lower your shoulders back down as you breathe out.
- Perform 10 repetitions.

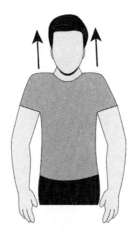

Figure 7-5 SHOULDER RAISES

#6 – **Chest/Shoulder Stretch** - hiking

This stretch improves your back, opens up your chest, and increases your shoulders' range of motion. It will also expand your lungs, so you get more oxygen when hiking.

- Stand tall with your feet together. Relax your arms and breath in.
- With your head upright and shoulders back and down, clasp your hands behind your back.
- Slowly turn your elbows inward as you extend your arms.
- Imagine grasping a ball behind you.
- With your chest out and chin in, lift your arms behind you until you feel a stretch.
- Hold for 10 to 15 seconds.

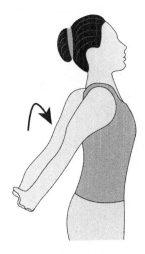

Figure 7-6 CHEST/SHOULDER STRETCH

#7 – **Tricep Stretch** - hiking

This stretch loosens up your arm muscles and opens up your shoulders. It's excellent for increasing upper body strength, preventing muscle tension and injury.

- Stand with feet shoulder-width apart.
- Raise your left arm and bend it at the elbow. Your elbow should be pointing upwards and with the arm behind your head.
- Grab the left elbow with your right hand and pull across until you feel the stretch in your upper arm.
- Hold this position for 10 to 15 seconds.
- Return to starting position, breath, switch sides and repeat.
- Hold again for 10 to 15 seconds. Perform 2 to 3 repetitions on each side.

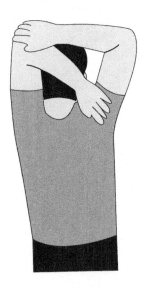

Figure 7-7 TRICEP STRETCH

#8 – Hip Flexor Stretch - hiking

This stretches your hip flexor muscles, which allow flexion on the hip joint. It will improve your mechanics when hiking and prevent injury and pain on the hips and lower back.

- Start by kneeling (as if you're proposing) with the left knee on the ground and the right knee pointing forward.
- Place both hands on your right knee in front of you for balance and support and straighten your upper body.
- Keep your upper body straight while holding your hands firmly on your right knee for support.
- Move forward slowly until you feel a stretch.
- Hold for 10 to 20 seconds.
- Return to starting position and switch legs.
- Repeat 3 to 4 times on both sides.

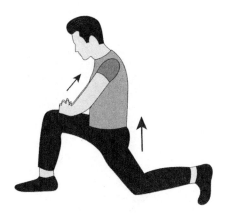

Figure 7-8 HIP FLEXOR STRETCH

#9 – **Calf Stretch** - hiking

This will stretch your gastrocnemius and soleus muscles which are taxed when hiking. It will help prevent calf injuries and pain.

- Stand in front of solid support – a wall makes for a good choice.
- Place your hands on the support.
- Place the left foot in front of you, leg bent.
- Your right leg should be straight behind you.
- Move your hips forward slowly until you feel a stretch in the calf of your right leg.
- Keep the right heel flat and toes pointing straight forward.
- Hold this position for 1o to 15 seconds.
- Switch legs and alternate for 3 repetitions.
- Ensure you don't bounce or hold your breath.

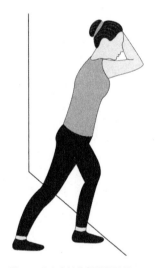

Figure 7-9 CALF STRETCH

#10 – **Partial Squats** - hiking

This exercise stretches your quads, hamstrings, Achilles, calves, and ankles. It improves your balance and mobility and helps prevent falls. It is a great exercise to help with endurance during hiking.

- Stand with feet shoulder-width apart.
- Place your hands on your hips for balance.
- Assume a bent knee position (quarter squat).
- Keep heels flat with toes pointing forward.
- Hold this position for 30 seconds.
- Repeat this exercise 3 times.

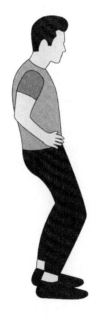

Figure 7-10 PARTIAL SQUATS

Golfing

GOLFING

The metallic "ping" of the driver's clubhead cleanly hitting the ball - is the sound that golfers love! This peaceful sport is loved by many and, although relatively slow and unhurried, is considered strenuous. The art of driving the ball down the fairway is all about using the right clubs and making the right decisions. It's also about the twists and pulls of the body as it goes through the physical motions of hitting the ball in a timely fashion. Many upper-body muscles in the chest, arms, and back go into mastering the perfect tee-off. This sport also requires extensive walking using muscles in the thighs and calves. Warming the muscles with simple stretching exercises is bound to help with those elusive birdies. Here are a few of the stretches that will improve your golfing abilities and even put a bit of advantage into your game!

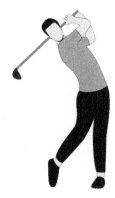

#1 – **Scarecrow Twists** - golfing

The twisting action helps improve your core strength, flexibility, stability, and spine mobility. It's good for your spine and will prepare your body to swing a golf club.

- Stand with your feet slightly wider than your shoulders.
- Place your golf club behind your neck onto your shoulders.
- Place both your arms over the golf club in a scarecrow position.
- Slightly bend your knees and inhale. On the exhale, twist to the right, pivoting on your left foot.
- Hold for 5 seconds, looking over your shoulder.
- Repeat on the other side, twisting to your left.
- Perform the twisting action 8 times on each side, breathing throughout.

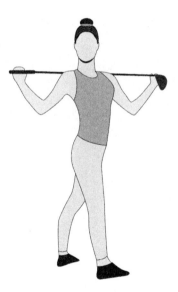

Figure 8-1 SCARECROW TWISTS

#2 – Neck Turns - golfing

This exercise stretches the sternocleidomastoid (SCM) muscle used when turning your head. It will improve your range of motion, make it easy to turn when playing and relieve neck pain.

- Stand in a neutral position.
- Place feet a little wider than shoulder width apart.
- Turn your face to one side to look over your shoulder.
- Hold that position for 5 to 10 seconds.
- Return to neutral position and turn to the other side.
- Hold for 5 to 10 seconds.
- Repeat 2 to 4 times on each side.

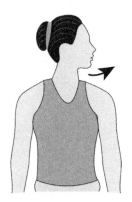

Figure 8-2 NECK TURNS

#3 – **Standing Abdominal Stretch** - golfing

This exercise opens up and loosens your core, back, and shoulders. It will help you get a better posture and address position when golfing.

- Reach your arms upward extending them overhead.
- Place your palms together.
- Extend your arms upwards and lean back slightly.
- Stay balanced through the stretch.
- Hold the stretch for 10 to 15 seconds.
- Inhale as you stretch up, exhale when lowering arms.
- Repeat 8 to 10 times.

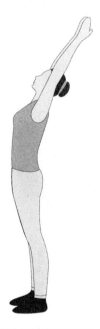

Figure 8-3 STANDING ABDOMINAL STRETCH

#4 – **Partial Squats** - golfing

This will stretch your quads, hamstrings, achilles, calves, and ankles. It will give you more balance and mobility and help prevent falls. It helps to establish a good stance for your most important tee-offs!

- Stand with feet shoulder-width apart.
- Place your hands to your sides and assume a bent knee position.
- Lower yourself to a quarter squat.
- Keep heels flat with toes pointing forward.
- Hold this position for 30 seconds.
- Stand up and rest for a few moments.
- Repeat the exercise another 2 times.

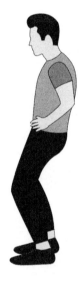

Figure 8-4 PARTIAL SQUATS

#5 – **Upward Wrist Flexor** - golfing

This exercise stretches the flexor carpi and biceps brachii muscles are responsible for wrist flexion, abduction, and forearm supination. It will increase your wrist flexibility and lower the risk of injuries like golfers' elbow.

- While standing, extend your arms out straight in front of you with palms facing downwards.
- Raise your arms to shoulder height and keep your elbows straight.
- Move up your fingers upwards toward your head and spread them while exhaling.
- Hold this position for 10 to 15 seconds.
- Brings your arms down and shake them out.
- Repeat another 3 times.

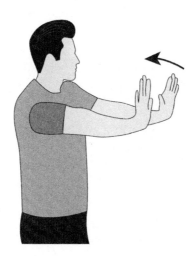

Figure 8-5 UPWARD WRIST FLEXOR

#6 – Downward Wrist Extensor - golfing

This exercise stretches your extensor and hand muscles which work together to extend the wrist. It stimulates and improves blood flow to the wrist area and prevents carpal tunnel injuries.

- While standing, extend your arms out straight in front of you with palms facing downwards.
- Raise your arms to shoulder height and keep your elbows straight.
- Curl your fingers down toward, and feel the stretch in your forearms
- Breathe while holding this position for 10 to 15 seconds.
- Bring your arms down and shake them out.
- Repeat at least another 2 times.

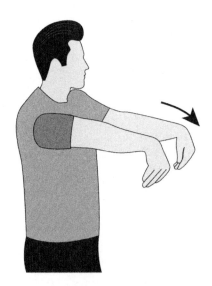

Figure 8-6 DOWNWARD WRIST EXTENSOR

#7 – **Side Stretch** - golfing

This exercise develops the flexibility of your arms, shoulders, and trunk muscles. It's excellent for improving upper body strength and preventing injury as you swing your club.

- While standing, raise your right hand and bend it behind your head.
- Grasp above the right elbow with your left hand.
- Pull to the left while leaning as far as you can.
- Hold this position for 5 to 10 seconds.
- Return to starting position.
- Switch hands and pull to the right.
- Repeat 3 to 5 times for both sides.

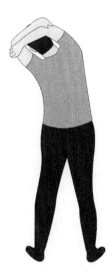

Figure 8-7 SIDE STRETCH

#8 – Ankle Circles - golfing

This exercise stretches the ankle, calf, and feet muscles. It will improve your flexibility, increase your ankles' stability and mobility, and prevent walking injuries. Keep your ankles strong and flexible with this motion.

- Stand upright with feet hip-width apart and arms by your sides.
- Hold on to something like a table for balance with your right hand and lift your left foot a few inches from the ground.
- Without moving your leg, rotate the left ankle in a clockwise direction.
- Perform 5 to 10 rotations and return to starting position.
- Switch legs and repeat.

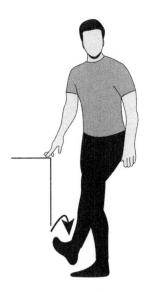

Figure 8-8 ANKLE CIRCLES

#9 – Calf Stretch - golfing

This will stretch the calf muscles taxed by walking and help prevent calf injuries and pain while moving around the course.

- Stand in front of a wall and lean on it with your forearms. Rest your head on your arms.
- Place the left foot in front of you, leg bent.
- Your right leg should be straight behind you.
- Move your hips forward slowly until you feel a stretch in the calf of your right leg.
- Keep the right heel flat and toes pointing straight forward.
- Hold this position for 1o to 15 seconds.
- Switch legs and alternate for 3 repetitions.
- Ensure you don't bounce or hold your breath.

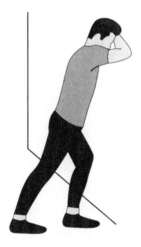

Figure 8-9 CALF STRETCH

#10 – **Seated Neck Stretch** - golfing

This is good for loosening up the neck and shoulders.

- Sit on a firm chair while keeping your back straight and your feet flat on the floor. Raise your hands and place them behind your head with fingers interlocked as if basking in the sun on the beach.
- Slowly ease your head backward into your hands and lift your face towards the ceiling.
- Breathe in deeply. As you exhale, lean your right elbow down toward the ground and your left elbow up toward the ceiling.
- You should feel a gentle but supported stretch in your neck.
- Hold that position (which is only slight, by the way) for two deep breaths and then slowly return to the starting position.
- Repeat this on the opposite side. Try to do at least four reps on each side.

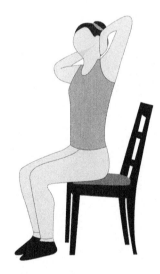

Figure 8-10 SEATED NECK STRETCH

#11 – Seated Back Bend - golfing

This stretch is good for the neck, spine, and back.

- Sit on a firm chair and position your feet flat on the floor with your back straight.
- Position your hands onto your lower back with fingers wrapped onto your hips.
- Push your hands into your hips/lower back and breathe in deeply.
- As you breathe out, push backward with your head and arch your back. Your chin should tilt upward, and your face should face the ceiling.
- Hold the arched position for the count of five deep breaths and then return to the starting position.
- Repeat this movement at least six times.

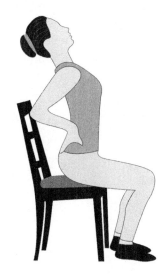

Figure 8-11 SEATED BACK BEND

Swimming

SWIMMING

This low-impact sport is a great way to burn calories and de-stress. It also provides a full-body workout while you are having fun. This means that all your muscles are engaged and working together to keep you afloat and moving through the water. Different swimming strokes require the use of specific muscles in both your arms and legs at the same time.

The repetitive swimming strokes and natural resistance provided by the water give your muscles a complete workout as though you were training at the gym. With so many muscles working at once, it makes sense to stretch and prevent any cramps and strain while swimming. Make a point of doing these stretches before you plunge into the pool.

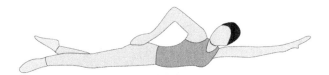

#1 – **Abdominal Stretch** - swimming

This exercise stretches your abdominals, latissimus dorsi, obliques, and biceps. It loosens your upper body and gets the muscles ready for swimming movements. Dive in knowing you're completely prepared.

- Reach your arms upward extending them overhead.
- Place your palms together.
- Extend your arms upwards and lean back slightly.
- Stay balanced through the stretch.
- Hold the stretch for 10 to 15 seconds.
- Inhale as you stretch up, exhale when lowering arms.
- Repeat 8 to 10 times.

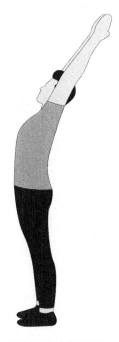

Figure 9-1 ABDOMINAL STRETCH

#2 - **Standing Side Stretch** - swimming

This exercise develops the flexibility of your arms, shoulders, and trunk muscles. It's excellent for improving upper body strength and preventing injury as you swim.

- Stand with feet a little wider than shoulder width.
- Raise your left hand and bend it behind your head.
- Grasp your left elbow with your right hand and grasp your right elbow with your left hand.
- Lean toward the right as far as you can.
- Hold this position for 5 to 10 seconds.
- Return to starting position.
- Switch hands and pull to the right.
- Repeat 3 to 5 times for both sides.

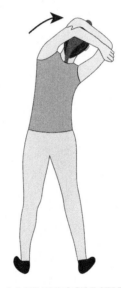

Figure 9-2 STANDING SIDE STRETCH

#3 – Cross Body Shoulder Stretch - swimming

This exercise targets the rotator cuff muscles to improve your range of motion. It will prevent pain and reduce the risk for injury while performing your swimming strokes.

- Stand with your feet hip-width apart.
- Put your left hand on your right shoulder.
- Cup your left elbow with your right hand.
- Roll your shoulders down and back as you gently pull your left elbow across your chest.
- Hold 10 to 30 seconds.
- Switch hands and repeat on the other side.
- Perform 3 to 4 sets of 8 repetitions on each side.

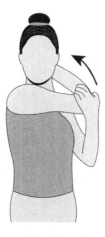

Figure 9-3 CROSS BODY SHOULDER STRETCH

#4 – Chest/Shoulder Stretch - swimming

This stretch improves your back, opens up your chest, and increases your shoulders' range of motion. It will also expand your lungs, so you get more oxygen underwater.

- Stand tall with your feet together.
- Relax your arms and breath in.
- With your head upright and shoulders back and down, clasp your hands behind your back.
- Slowly turn your elbows inward as you extend your arms.
- Imagine grasping a ball behind you.
- With your chest out and chin up, lift your arms behind you until you feel a stretch.
- Hold for 10 to 15 seconds.
- Repeat the exercise 3 times.

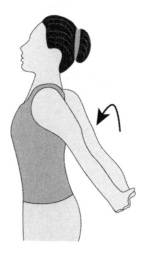

Figure 9-4 CHEST/SHOULDER STRETCH

5 – **Partial Crunches** - swimming

This exercise targets the abdominal muscles to improve lower back health and strengthen the core. The core plays a significant role in swimming and how well you move in the water.

- Lie flat on your back with your knees bent and feet flat on the floor.
- Place your hands behind your head for support.
- This is the start position.
- Lift from your waist towards your knees, contracting your abdominal muscles as you curl your spine into a crunch position.
- Breathe out as you perform the crunch and hold for a few seconds.
- Return to the start position and repeat 4 to 6 times.

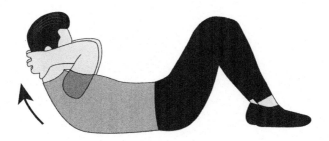

Figure 9-5 PARTIAL CRUNCHES

6 – **Seated Torso Stretch** - swimming

This exercise stretches your hip abductors, latissimus dorsi, erector spinae, and oblique muscles. It will improve your rotational motions, flexibility and improve core strength.

- Sit on the ground with the left leg forward and straight.
- Cross the left leg over the right while sitting erect.
- Slowly rotate the upper body to the left and look over your left shoulder.
- Reach across the left leg with your right arm and push the left leg to your right.
- Use the left arm for support by placing it on the ground.
- Hold this position for 10 to 15 seconds.
- Switch sides and repeat by crossing and turning in the opposite direction.
- Perform 5 to 10 repetitions on each side.

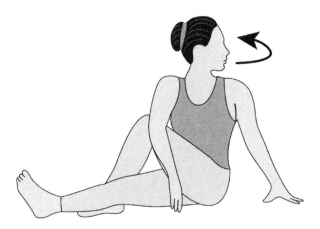

Figure 9-6 SEATED TORSO STRETCH

7 - **Hip Flexor Stretch** - swimming

This stretches your hip flexor muscles, which allow flexion on the hip joint. It will improve your mechanics when swimming and prevent injury and pain on the hips and lower back.

- Start by kneeling as if you're proposing, the left knee on the ground and the right knee pointing forward.
- Place both hands on the ground for balance and support.
- Lean forward slowly while pressing downwards with your hips until you feel a stretch on your right thigh.
- Hold for 10 to 20 seconds.
- Return to starting position and switch legs.
- Repeat 3 to 4 times on both sides.

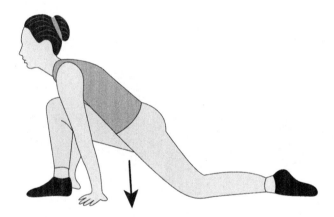

Figure 9-7 HIP FLEXOR STRETCH

#8 – Deep Body-Weight Squat - swimming

This exercise stretches your hamstrings, glutes, calf muscles, and quadriceps. It's excellent for increasing mobility and strength and improving your functional movement and lower back and pelvic stability.

- Position your feet shoulder-width apart and stand firm.
- Slowly squat down as if you're sitting in a chair.
- Your ankles, knees, and hips should bend in unison while your back remains straight.
- To improve and maintain balance at the lowest depth, use your fingertips to touch the floor in front of you.
- Your feet should remain flat on the ground for the entire movement.
- Hold this position for as long as you can, starting with at least 30 seconds to one minute.

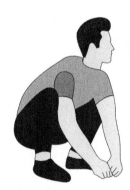

Figure 9-8 DEEP BODY-WIEGHT SQUAT

#9 – Calf Stretch - swimming

This will stretch your gastrocnemius and soleus muscles and help prevent calf injuries and pain.

- Stand in front of a wall and lean on it with your forearms.
- Rest your head on your arms.
- Place the left foot in front of you, leg bent.
- Your right leg should be straight behind you.
- Move your hips forward slowly until you feel a stretch in the calf of your right leg.
- Keep the left heel flat and toes pointing straight forward.
- Hold this position for 1o to 15 seconds.
- Switch legs and alternate for 3 repetitions. Ensure you don't bounce or hold your breath.

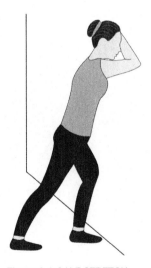

Figure 9-9 CALF STRETCH

#10 – Back Leg Raises - swimming

This stretch strengthens the lower back, making it less prone to injuries.

- Stand up straight behind a chair.
- Hold on to chair for stability.
- With a slow movement, lift either leg straight back without bending your knees or pointing your toes.
- Keep your leg straight back for three seconds and then return to the start position.
- Repeat this stretch ten times and then switch to the other leg.

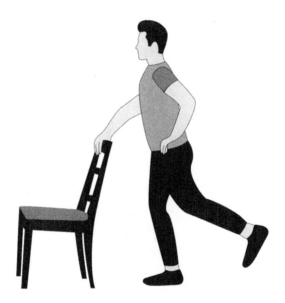

Figure 9-10 BACK LEG RAISES

Tennis Pickleball

TENNIS & PICKLEBALL

Both tennis and pickleball are fun, friendly ways to socialize while working out. Taking your stress out on the ball with your racket or paddle goes a long way to helping you de-stress and exercise at that same time. Much like tennis, pickleball entails swotting a ball over the net while dashing madly around the court, lunging to bat the ball, or stretching to tap it back towards your opponent. This type of arm movement engages a host of muscles in the back, forearm, and shoulders. Not to mention the muscles used in your legs while running up and down. By incorporating the following stretching routine before a healthy game of tennis or pickleball, you can prevent shoulder pain, tennis elbow, and calf strain.

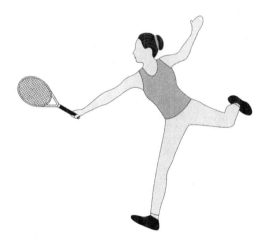

#1 – **Hip Flexor Stretch** - tennis & pickleball

This stretches your hip flexor muscles, which allow flexion on the hip joint. It will improve your mechanics when moving and prevent injury and pain on the hips and lower back.

- Start by kneeling (as if you're proposing) with the left knee on the ground and the right knee pointing forward.
- Place both hands on your right knee in front of you for balance and support and straighten your upper body.
- Keep your upper body straight while holding your hands firmly on your right knee for support.
- Move forward slowly until you feel a stretch.
- Hold for 10 to 20 seconds.
- Return to starting position and switch legs.
- Repeat 3 to 4 times on both sides.

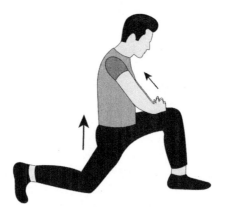

Figure 10-1 HIP FLEXOR STRETCH

#2 – **Deep Body Weight Squat** - tennis & pickleball

This exercise stretches your hamstrings, glutes, calf muscles, and quadriceps. It's excellent for increasing mobility and strength and improving your functional movement and lower back and pelvic stability.

- Position your feet shoulder-width apart and stand firm.
- Slowly squat down as if you're sitting in a chair.
- Your ankles, knees, and hips should bend in unison while your back remains straight.
- To improve and maintain balance at the lowest depth, use your fingertips to touch the floor in front of you.
- Your feet should remain flat on the ground for the entire movement.
- Hold this position for as long as you can, starting with at least 30 seconds to one minute.

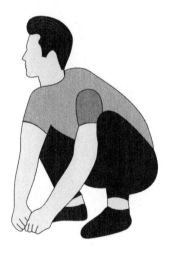

Figure 10-2 DEEP BODY WIEGHT SQUAT

#3 – **Shoulder Shrugs** - tennis & pickleball

This exercise stretches your trapezius muscles which control shoulder blade, neck, and upper back movement. Toned and robust trapezius will improve the efficiency and safety of your sports movements.

- Stand with your feet shoulder-width apart and flat on the floor.
- Slightly bend your knees, so they line up with your toes.
- Keep your chin up, neck straight, and face straight ahead.
- Inhale and slowly bring your shoulders as high up towards your ears as you can.
- Hold this position for 5 seconds.
- Lower your shoulders back down and exhale.
- Perform 3 sets of 10 repetitions.

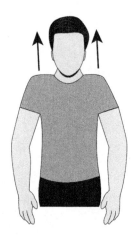

Figure 10-3 SHOULDER SHRUGS

#4 - Cross Body Shoulder Stretch - tennis & pickleball

This exercise targets the rotator cuff muscles to improve your range of motion, prevent pain and reduce the risk for injury while playing.

- Stand with your feet hip-width apart.
- Put your right hand on your left shoulder.
- Cup your right elbow with your left hand.
- Roll your shoulders down and back as you gently pull your right elbow across your chest.
- Hold 10 to 30 seconds.
- Switch hands and repeat on the other side.
- Perform 2 - 3 sets of 6 repetitions on each side.

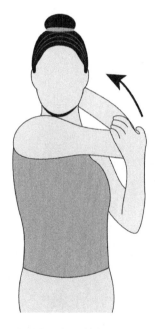

Figure 10-4 CROSS BODY SHOULDER STRETCH

#5 – **Standing Abdominal Stretch** - tennis & pickleball

This exercise stretches your abdominals, latissimus dorsi, obliques, and biceps. It loosens your upper body and gets the muscles ready for sports movements.

- Reach your arms upward over your head.
- Hold your palms together.
- Extend your arms upwards.
- While keeping your balance, slightly lean backward.
- Hold the stretch for 10 to 15 seconds.
- Inhale as you stretch up, exhale when lowering arms.
- Repeat 8 to 10 times.

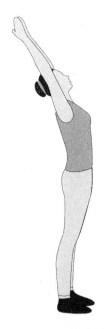

Figure 10-5 STANDING ABDOMINAL STRETCH

#6 – Tricep Stretch - tennis & pickleball

This stretch loosens up your arm muscles and opens up your shoulders. It's excellent for increasing upper body strength, preventing muscle tension and injury.

- Stand with feet shoulder-width apart.
- Raise your left arm and bend it at the elbow. Your elbow should be pointing upwards and with the arm behind your head.
- Grab the left elbow with your right hand and pull across as far as comfortable.
- Hold this position for 10 to 15 seconds.
- Return to starting position, breath, switch sides and repeat.
- Hold again for 10 to 15 seconds.
- Perform 2 to 3 repetitions on each side.

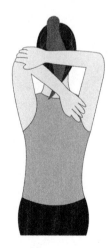

Figure 10-6 TRICEP STRETCH

7 – **Wall Rotation Stretch** - tennis & pickleball

This exercise stretches your trunk muscles for improved thoracic spine mobility. Optimal mobility of the thoracic spine is vital for performing well and preventing muscle and joint injuries when playing tennis.

- Stand at arm's length and place palms on the wall.
- Position your left foot forward and your right foot back.
- Rotate your torso to the left and use your hands to create more rotation.
- You should feel a stretch around your torso and tension behind the left shoulder blade as you retract that shoulder.
- Hold this position for 30 seconds.
- Return to starting position and switch sides.
- Repeat 3 times on each side.

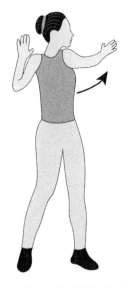

Figure 10-7 WALL ROTATION STRETCH

8 – **Quad Stretch** - tennis & pickleball

This exercise stretches the quadriceps and anterior tibialis. It helps your quads gain and maintain flexibility and warms up the anterior tibialis to ensure you don't trip over when walking or running.

- Stand at arm's length from a sturdy object with your left foot on flat ground.
- Place your right hand on the solid object for support and balance
- Bend your right leg up towards your buttocks.
- Grasp the top of your right foot with your left hand.
- Pull your foot in towards your right buttock, ensuring your knee is pointing towards the ground.
- Hold this position for 10 to 15 seconds.
- Switch sides and repeat 3 - 4 times each side.

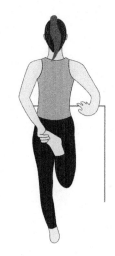

Figure 10-8 QUAD STRETCH

#9 – Partial Squat - tennis & pickleball

This will stretch your quads, hamstrings, achilles, calves, and ankles. It will give you more balance and mobility and help prevent falls.

- Position your feet shoulder-width apart and stand firm.
- Place your hands to your sides and assume a bent knee position (about a quarter squat).
- Keep heels flat with toes pointing forward.
- Hold this position for 20 - 30 seconds.
- Repeat the exercise 3 times.

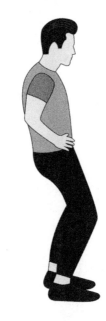

Figure 10-9 PARTIAL SQUAT

#10 – Calf Stretch - tennis, pickleball

This will stretch your gastrocnemius and soleus muscles and help prevent calf injuries and pain.

- Stand in front of a wall and lean on it with your forearms. Rest your head on your arms.
- Place the right foot in front of you, leg bent.
- Your left leg should be straight behind you.
- Move your hips forward slowly until you feel a stretch in the calf of your left leg.
- Keep the left heel flat and toes pointing straight forward.
- Hold this position for 10 to 15 seconds.
- Switch legs and alternate for 3 repetitions.
- Ensure you don't bounce or hold your breath.

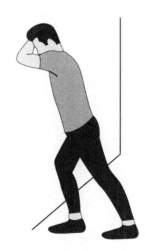

Figure 10-10 CALF STRETCH

#11 – Seated Neck Stretch - tennis & pickleball

This is good for loosening up the neck and shoulders.

- Sit on a firm chair while keeping your back straight and your feet flat on the floor. Raise your hands and place them behind your head with fingers interlocked as if basking in the sun on the beach.
- Slowly ease your head backward into your hands and lift your face towards the ceiling.
- Breathe in deeply. As you exhale, lean your right elbow down toward the ground and your left elbow up toward the ceiling.
- You should feel a gentle but supported stretch in your neck.
- Hold that position (which is only slight, by the way) for two deep breaths and then slowly return to the starting position.
- Repeat this on the opposite side. Try to do at least four reps on each side.

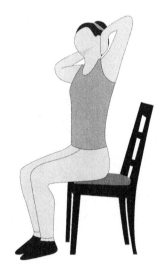

Figure 10-11 SEATED NECK STRETCH

#12 – **Forward Lunge** - tennis & pickleball

Forward lunges are a great stretching and strength exercise of the largest muscle group in the lower half of the body: the quads, hamstrings and calves. Other areas that will be engaged are the back, the core, and the glutes.

- Stand upright, look directly ahead, with your feet shoulder-width apart. Your toes should be facing forward.
- Move your right leg forward to take a big step.
- Lower your body until your right thigh is parallel to the floor.
- Press your right heel to drive back up to the upright starting position.
- Repeat the same movement on the left side, then alternate each side 10 times.

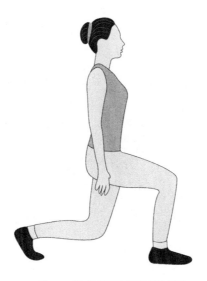

Figure 10-12 FORWARD LUNGE

Cycling

CYCLING

Zipping down those country roads or speeding along the suburbs, cycling has to be one of the most popular sports for people of all ages, including those of us over fifty. It's exhilarating feeling the wind in your hair and the sun on your face. The main muscle groups exercised while cycling can be found in your legs, namely the quadriceps and hamstrings. However, there is also a lot of work being done by your butt, the gluteus maximus. In addition, the back and abdomen muscles help to keep your upper body balanced. Stretching these muscles using the routine below reduces the risk of repetitive strain injuries, aches, and pains from being in one position.

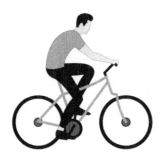

1 – **Knee to Chest Stretch** - cycling

This exercise stretches your hip flexors, quadriceps, glutes, and lower back. It will help improve the strength, flexibility, and mobility of your back and hips.

- Lie on your back with arms straight beside your body.
- Keep your legs straight and the knees and feet together.
- Bring the left leg straight back towards your head and leave the right leg at the starting position.
- Bring your arms up and grab the bent leg under the knees.
- Pull it gradually to your chest.
- Hold this position for 10 to 15 seconds.
- Slowly return to the starting position and switch to the right leg.
- Repeat 3 to 4 times on each side.

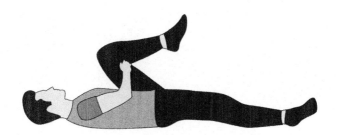

Figure 11-1 KNEE TO CHEST STRETCH

#2 – **Hip Flexor Stretch** - cycling

This exercise stretches the hip flexor muscles, which allow flexion on your hip joint. It will improve your mechanics and prevent injury and pain on the hips and lower back.

- Start in a standing position.
- Take a big step forward with your left leg like you're making an extended lunge.
- Plant your left foot firmly on the ground.
- Your right knee should be resting on the floor.
- Lower your right hip until you feel a stretch without changing position. Place your hands on the floor to avoid overextension or putting too much weight on your hips.
- Hold for 10 to 15 seconds.
- Return to starting position and switch legs.
- Repeat 2 to 3 times on each leg.

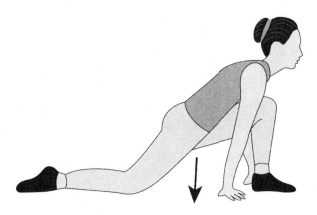

Figure 11-2 HIP FLEXOR STRETCH

#3 – Seated Groin Stretch - cycling

This exercise stretches the erector spinae and hip adductor muscles. This improves your stability while making serves and groundstrokes and prevents groin injuries from rapid direction changes.

- Get into a seated position.
- Bend your knees and bring your soles together.
- Hold your feet with your hands.
- Exhale and lean forward at the waist for a deeper stretch. Allow your chest to fall as close to the floor as possible.
- Hold for 20 to 30 seconds.
- Release and repeat 3 times.

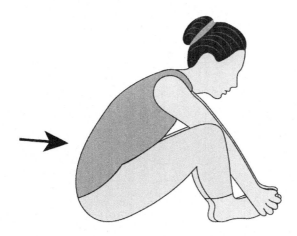

Figure 11-3 SEATED GROIN STRETCH

#4 – **Seated Hip Stretch** - cycling

This exercise stretches your hip abductors, latissimus dorsi, erector spinae, and oblique muscles. It will improve your rotational motions, flexibility and improve core strength.

- Sit on the ground with the right leg forward and straight.
- Cross the left leg over the right while sitting erect.
- Slowly rotate the upper body to the left and look over your left shoulder.
- Reach across the left leg with your right arm and push the left leg to your right.
- Use the left arm for support by placing it on the ground.
- Hold this position for 10 to 15 seconds.
- Switch sides and repeat by crossing and turning in the opposite direction.
- Perform 5 to 10 repetitions on each side.

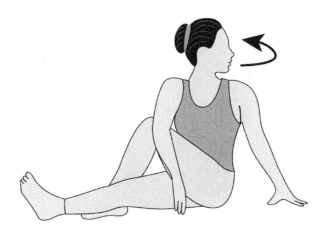

Figure 11-4 SEATED HIP STRETCH

#5 – **Partial Crunch** - cycling

This exercise targets the abdominal muscles to improve lower back health and strengthen the core. A strong core improves your balance and functional movements.

- Lie flat on your back with your knees bent and feet flat on the floor.
- Place your hands behind your head for support. This is the start position.
- Lift from your waist towards your knees, contracting your abdominal muscles as you curl your spine into a crunch position.
- Breathe out as you perform the crunch and hold for a few seconds.
- Return to the start position and repeat 4 to 6 times.

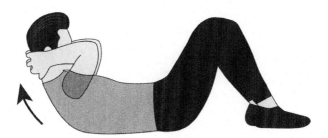

Figure 11-5 PARTIAL CRUNCH

6 – **Calf Stretch** - cycling

This will stretch your gastrocnemius and soleus muscles and help prevent calf injuries and pain.

- Stand in front of a wall and lean on it with your forearms.
- Rest your head on your arms.
- Place the left foot in front of you, leg bent.
- Your right leg should be straight behind you.
- Move hips slowly forward until you feel a stretch in your calf.
- Keep the right heel flat and toes pointing straight forward.
- Hold this position for 10 to 15 seconds.

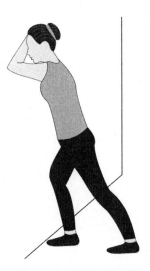

Figure 11-6 CALF STRETCH

#7 – **Quad Stretch** - cycling

This exercise stretches the quadriceps and anterior tibialis. It will help you develop and maintain flexibility and control. It also helps in making accelerated movements.

- Stand upright with feet hip-width apart.
- Hold on to a table for balance with your right hand.
- Lift your right leg by bending it up towards your buttocks.
- Grasp the top of your right foot with your left hand.
- Pull your foot in towards your right buttock, ensuring your knee is pointing towards the ground.
- Hold this position for 1o to 15 seconds.
- Switch sides and repeat 3 to 4 times on each side.

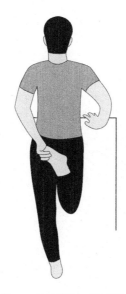

Figure 11-7 QUAD STRETCH

#8 – Deep Body-Weight Squat - cycling

This exercise stretches your hamstrings, glutes, calf muscles, and quadriceps. It's excellent for increasing mobility and strength and improving your functional movement and lower back and pelvic stability.

- Stand with your feet shoulder-width apart.
- Slowly squat down as if you're sitting in a chair.
- Your ankles, knees, and hips should bend in unison while your back remains straight.
- If needed, maintain your balance with your fingers touching the floor in front of you.
- The heels of your feet should remain flat on the ground
- Hold this squat stance for as long as you can, starting with at least 30 seconds to one minute and then relax.

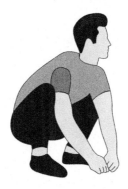

Figure 11-8 DEEP BODY-WEIGHT SQUAT

9 – **Hamstring Stretch** - cycling

This stretches the hamstrings, gluteal, and erector spinal muscles to improve your performance and flexibility while helping prevent tightness and pain.

- Stand with your feet hip-width apart and knees slightly bent.
- Bend forward and reach towards your toes.
- Keep your head up and legs straight.
- Hold this position for 10 to 15 seconds.
- Steadily breathe in and out throughout.

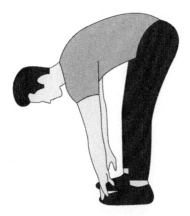

Figure 11-9 HAMSTRING STRETCH

10 – **Back Arch Stretch** - cycling

This stretch helps to relieve tension in your lower back and loosen up any tightness. At the same time it strengthens your back, hips, chest and shoulders. The aim of this exercise is to promote and improve mobility and increase your flexibility.

- Start positioned on the floor with your hands and knees hip-width apart.
- Arch the back, drawing your belly button up toward your spine while keeping your hands at shoulder-width apart.
- Hold for a brief second.
- Slowly relax the muscles allowing the stomach to naturally fall toward the floor, while exhaling. Keep your shoulders and hips in the very same position.
- Return to the starting position and repeat this motion a total of 10 times.

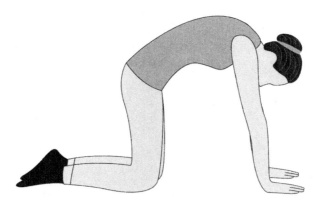

Figure 11-10 BACK ARCH STRETCH

Now that you're well on your way to building strength and flexibility, you have to spend some time maintaining it. Chapter seven: *Daily Tips for Staying Flexible* provides you with all the ins and outs of maintaining your developing strength, flexibility and mobility.

7

DAILY TIPS FOR STAYING FLEXIBLE

Something we have noticed many 50+ers do is get all excited about getting fit, flexible and fully mobile again, put in the work, and then suddenly stop because they've reached a goal or they're feeling great. The problem with this is that your newfound fitness and health will steadily decline, and suddenly you'll be back at square one again. Let's face it; square one is not somewhere you want to end up when you're heading past the 50 goal post. Believe it or not, stretching and other forms of exercise will not always be hard.

THE SECRETS TO STICKING WITH IT

The more you do it, the easier it will get. But there's a danger that comes with that, and the danger is called complacency. We cannot put enough emphasis on just how important it is to make your stretching part of your daily routine. You should be stretching to give your muscles a workout and stretching to maintain the progress you've already made. It may sound like a lot of stretching, but it's really not. Once you make it part of your life, it will become a natural thing to do – and trust us; your body will thank you for it.

Here's the secret to staying flexible, mobile, and strong forever: stretch every day. Simple, right? We think so! You probably don't want to embark on a 30-minute workout session if you're having a down day or running around after the grandkids without a minute to spare. If you can't do your regular fitness routine in scenarios where you should at least spend some time doing simple stretches for maintenance, and you can even do these with the grandkids, they might even find them fun and want to join in!

Stretching helps prime the muscles for movement, make you less prone to fall accidents and the associated injuries, and ensure that you manage to hang onto your independence. You know what *they* say, right? It can take you around three weeks to form a habit or break it, so just by dedicating yourself to doing some stretching every day for 21 days, you can make it become part of your life. You might just become addicted!

Without much further ado, let's go over a few simple daily stretches in the next few pages that will go a long way towards maintaining your strength, flexibility, and mobility.

15 Min Routine

THE 15-MINUTE ROUTINE

Try to set some time aside (consistently) for a daily 15-minute routine. 15 minutes of stretching qualifies as a mini workout, so try slot these stretches into your day whenever you can. This routine will take all of fifteen minutes when you do all stretches as explained in the following descriptions. Let's go!

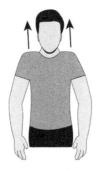

#1 SHOULDER RAISES

#1 - Shoulder Raises Shoulder raises are similar to a shrug except slow and intentional. This stretch increases shoulder mobility and brings more flexibility to the back and neck. Bring your shoulders up as far as they can go without hurting, this is a dramatic shrug. Hold this shrug stance for 10 seconds, and then relax your shoulders. Repeat 3 to 4 times.

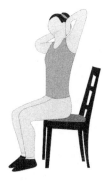

#2 SEATED NECK STRETCH

#2 – Seated Neck Stretch Sit on a firm chair while keeping your back straight and your feet flat on the floor. Clasp your hands behind your head. Slowly ease your head backward into your hands and lift your face towards the ceiling. Breathe in deeply. As you exhale, lean your right elbow down toward the ground and your left elbow up toward the ceiling. Hold that position for two deep breaths. Repeat four reps on each side.

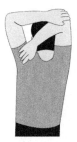

#3 TRICEP STRETCH

#3 – Tricep Stretch Stand with your feet hip-width apart. Bend your knees slightly. Raise your right arm in the air and bend your elbow so that your lower hand drops behind your head. Using your left hand, slowly push your right elbow downwards. Hold this stretch for 10 to 15 seconds. Repeat the arm stretch with the opposite arm. Do at least 2 of these arm stretches on each side.

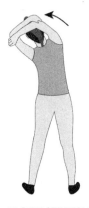

#4 SIDE STRETCH

#4 – Side Stretch Raise your arms above your head with arms shoulder-width apart. Bend your elbows so that each palm now touches the elbow of the opposite arm. Tighten your abdominal muscles, and then with a straight back bend slightly to the left side. Hold this stretch for 5 to 10 seconds. Do at least 2 stretches on each side.

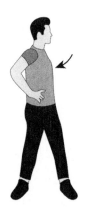

#5 TORSO ROTATIONS

#5 – Torso Rotations Stand with your feet shoulder-width apart, and then bend your knees slightly. Position your hands on your hips and then slowly and gently twist your upper body to the left while looking over your shoulder. Hold that twisted stretch for 10 to 15 seconds and then repeat the stretch on the right side. Repeat this stretch twice on each side. It's important to focus on a slow, steady, and fluid movement.

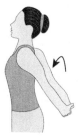

#6 CHEST/SHOULDER STRETCH

#6 – Chest/Shoulder Stretch Stand tall with your feet together. Relax your arms and breath in. With your head upright and shoulders back and down, clasp your hands behind your back. Slowly turn your elbows inward as you extend your arms. Imagine grasping a ball behind you. With your chest out and chin in, lift your arms behind you until you feel a stretch. Hold for 10 to 15 seconds. Repeat twice.

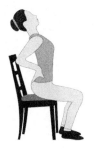

#7 SEATED BACK BEND

#7 – Seated Back Bend Sit on a firm chair and position your feet flat on the floor with your back straight. Position your hands onto your lower back with fingers facing downward. Push your hands into your hips/lower back and breathe in deeply. Push backward with your head and arch your back. Your chin should tilt upward. Hold the arched position for the count of five deep breaths and then return to the starting position. Repeat this movement six times.

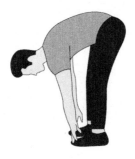

#8 HAMSTRING STRETCH

#8 – Hamstring Stretch Stand up with your back straight and with your feet shoulder-width apart. Slowly bend your torso forward at the hips while keeping your knees bent slightly. Relax your arm and neck as you bend forward until the point when you feel slight stretching in the backs of your legs. Hold for 10 seconds. Repeat 4 times.

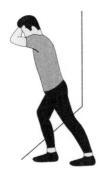

#9 CALF STRETCH

#9 – Calf Stretch Do this standing in front of a wall. Rest your head on your arms. Place the right foot in front of you, leg bent. Your left leg should be straight out behind you. Slowly move your hips forward until you start to feel a stretch in the calf muscle of your left leg. Keep the left heel flat and toes pointing straight forward. Hold for 10 seconds. Switch legs.

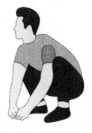

#10 FULL SQUAT

#10 – Full Squat Position your feet shoulder-width apart. Slowly squat down. Your ankles, knees, and hips should bend in unison while your back remains straight. To maintain balance at the lowest depth, hold your fingers down in front of you, keeping feet flat on the ground. Hold for 30 - 60 second. Repeat this stretch 2 more times.

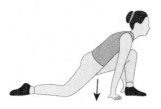

#11 HIP FLEXOR STRETCH

#11 – Hip Flexor Stretch While in a standing position, take a deep step forward using your right foot like you're making a lunge. Position your right foot firmly on the ground at a 90-degree angle. Your left knee should be resting gently on the floor. Lower your left hip until you feel a stretch. Place your hands on the floor to avoid overextension. Hold for 10 to 15 seconds. Switch legs and repeat 3 times.

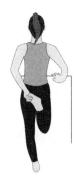

#12 QUAD STRETCH

#12 – Quad Stretch Place your left hand flat onto the wall in front of you and stand on your right foot - bend your left leg at the knee. Grip your left foot with your right hand and gently stretch and hold for 5 – 10 seconds. Repeat with the other leg. Complete 2 stretches on each leg.

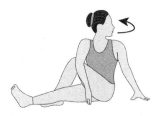

#13 SEATED TRUNK STRETCH

#13 – Seated Trunk Stretch Sit down on the floor, keeping your left leg bent and the other extended. Cross the left leg over your right leg and twist your trunk to the right. Place your left elbow onto your left knee to help your stretch. The idea is to slowly extend the muscles so you can turn and look behind you. Repeat this stretch 3 times on each side.

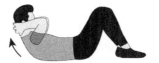

#14 NECK TENSION REDUCTION

#14 – Neck Tension Reduction This stretches your upper spine and neck. Lie on the floor and lock your hands behind your head. Slowly pull your head forward until you feel the stretch. Hold for 5 to 10 seconds and then repeat.

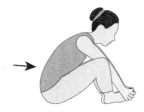

#15 BUTTERFLY STRETCH

#15 – Butterfly Stretch Sit on the floor with your feet facing each other. Your legs should not be crossed but should have knees bent and pulled as close to you as you can manage. Hold onto your toes and gently push down on your legs with your arms for 5 seconds and then relax. Repeat twice.

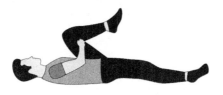

#16 HIP STRETCH

#16 – Hip Stretch Firmly pull your right leg up toward your chest with both hands behind your knee while lying flat on your back. Keep your head on the mat. Next, try to pull your leg toward the opposite shoulder to help stretch the outside of your hip. Hold for 5 seconds, then release. Repeat on the opposite leg.

10 Min Routine

THE 10-MINUTE ROUTINE

If you find yourself with 10 minutes of extra time, you should try to squeeze in this routine. Perhaps while you're waiting for the grand-kids to wake up for a nap or while you're waiting for your evening meal to cook you will find ten minutes available. During this routine, you have more time to go through a few more stretches. Some people find this routine the happy medium.

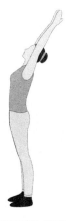

#1 ABDOMINAL STRETCH

#1 – Abdominal Stretch Stand feet together and raise your arms overhead. Hold your palms together like you just clapped your hands. Lean slightly back as you lift your chest up and arch your back. Keep your arms extended as you move them behind your head. Hold for 10 to 15 seconds and return to start. Rest for 15 seconds and repeat 3 more times.

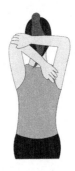

#2 TRICEP STRETCH

#2 – Tricep Stretch Stand with your feet hip-width apart. Bend your knees slightly. Raise your left arm in the air and bend your elbow so that your hand drops behind your head. Using your right hand, slowly push your left elbow across. Hold this stretch for 10 to 15 seconds. Repeat the arm stretch with the opposite arm. Do at least 2 of these arm stretches on each side.

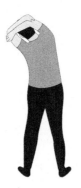

#3 SIDE STRETCH

#3 – Side Stretch Raise your arms above your head with arms shoulder-width apart and arms facing each other. Bend your elbows so that each palm now touches the elbow of the opposite arm. Tighten your abdominal muscles, and then with a straight back and holding firmly onto your elbows, bend slightly to the left side. Feel the muscle stretch on the opposite side and in your shoulders. Hold this stretch for 5 to 10 seconds. Do at least 2 stretches on each side.

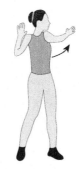

#4 TORSON ROTATION

#4 – Torso Rotation Stand with your feet shoulder-width apart, and bend your knees slightly. Slowly and gently twist your upper body to the left while looking over your shoulder. Do not push too far. Hold that twisted stretch for 5 to 10 seconds and then repeat the stretch on the right side. You may be tempted to bounce during this exercise, but it's important to focus on a slow, steady, and fluid movement.

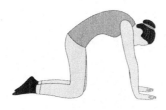

#7 BACK ARCH

#5 – Back Arch Start positioned on the floor with your hands and knees hip-width apart. Arch the back, drawing your belly button up toward your spine while keeping your hands at shoulder-width apart. Hold for a brief second. Slowly relax the muscles allowing the stomach to naturally fall toward the floor, while exhaling. Keep your shoulders and hips in the very same position. Return to the starting position and repeat this motion a total of 10 times.

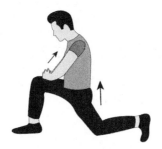

#6 HIP FLEXOR STRETCH

#6 – Hip Flexor Stretch While in a standing position, take a deep step forward using your right foot like you're making a lunge. Position your right foot firmly on the ground at a 90-degree angle. Place your hands on your right leg for stability. Your left knee should be resting gently on the floor. Lower your left hip until you feel a stretch. Hold for 10 to 15 seconds. Switch legs and repeat 3 times.

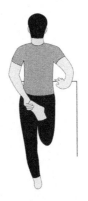

#7 QUAD STRETCH

#7 – Quad Stretch Place your left hand flat onto the wall in front of you and stand on your right foot - bend your left leg at the knee. Grip your left foot with your right hand and gently stretch and hold for 5 – 10 seconds. Repeat with the other leg. Complete 2 stretches on each leg.

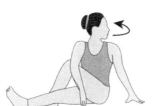

#8 SEATED TRUNK STRETCH

#8 – Seated Trunk Stretch Sit down on the floor, keeping your left leg bent and the other extended. Cross the left leg over your right leg and twist your trunk to the right. Place your left elbow onto your left knee to help your stretch. The idea is to slowly extend the muscles so you can turn and look behind you. Repeat this stretch 3 times on each side.

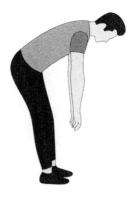

#5 LOWER BACK STRETCH

#5 – Lower Back Stretch Stand with feet shoulder length apart. Bend slowly forward from the hips. Keep your knees slightly bent so your lower back is not stressed. Relax your arms and neck and hold the extension until you feel the muscles in the back of your legs. Maintain stretch 5 to 10 seconds, then repeat 3 times.

5 Min Routine

THE 5-MINUTE ROUTINE

Yup, you read right! You only need to free up around five minutes to get a few stretches in each day. Of course, five-minute routines aren't going to be particularly action-packed or demanding, but they're certainly effective.

These are maintenance stretches rather than gearing up for a particular activity. However, we still advise you to use the full stretching routines in chapter 5 when doing a cardio or sports activity. We encourage you to try out each of the following stretches as you read through them, just to get a feel for them.

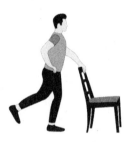

#1 BACK LEG RAISES

#1 - Back Leg Raises This stretch strengthens the lower back, making it less prone to injuries. Stand up straight behind a chair. With a slow movement, lift your left leg straight back without bending your knees or pointing your toes. Keep your leg straight back for three seconds and then return to the start position. Repeat this stretch ten times and then switch to the right leg.

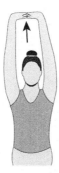

#2 OVERHEAD STRETCH

#2 – Overhead Stretch Reach your arms upward and extend them over your head with your palms together. Hold the overhead stretch for 10 to 15 seconds, and then bring your arms down. Inhale as you stretch up and exhale when you bring your arms down. Repeat 4 times.

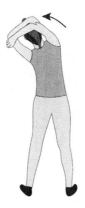

#3 SIDE STRETCH

#3 – Side Stretch Raise your arms above your head with arms shoulder-width apart and arms facing each other. Bend your elbows so that each palm now touches the elbow of the opposite arm. Tighten your abdominal muscles, and then with a straight back and holding firmly onto your elbows, bend slightly to the left side. Feel the muscle stretch on the opposite side and in your shoulders. Hold this stretch for 5 to 10 seconds. Do at least 2 stretches on each side.

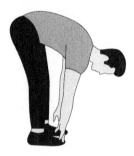

#4 HAMSTRING STRETCH

#4 – Hamstring Stretch Stand up with your back straight and with your feet shoulder-width apart. Slowly bend your torso forward at the hips while keeping your knees bent slightly. Relax your arm and neck as you bend forward until the point when you feel slight stretching in the backs of your legs. Hold for 10 seconds. Repeat 4 times.

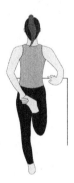

#5 QUAD STRETCH

#5 – Quad Stretch Place your left hand flat onto the wall in front of you and stand on your right foot - bend your left leg at the knee. Grip your left foot with your right hand and gently stretch and hold for 5 – 10 seconds. Repeat with the other leg. Complete 2 stretches on each leg.

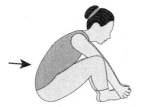

#6 BUTTERFLY STRETCH

#6 – Butterfly Stretch Sit on the floor with your feet facing each other. Your legs should not be crossed but should have knees bent and pulled as close to you as you can manage. Hold onto your toes and gently push down on your legs with your arms for 5 seconds and then relax. Repeat twice.

HOW TO STRETCH AT WORK/DESK

If you still spend time at work or behind a desk, the chances are that you're suffering with aches, pains, and discomforts. We spend years hunching over, leaning forward, and generally wreaking havoc on our postures, and then in our older years, we spend just as much time surprised and overwhelmed by the discomforts plaguing our bodies. The good news is that even if you already have pain, you can mitigate the pain by carrying out a few clever stretches.

We have found stretch bands quite helpful for stretching while at a desk. You can simply slip the stretch band below your feet and give your arms a mini stretch workout. If you want to focus on your lower back and hips, sit on the edge of your seat and position your feet below your knees. Cross one ankle over the opposite knee and gently pull your body forward.

Another great stretch for your back is to turn sideways in your chair. Hold the back of the chair, gently twist the front of your body toward the back of your chair. Then, slowly switch to the opposite side.

Your shoulders can also get tight from typing and fiddling around on the internet. You can loosen your shoulders and ease pain with a simple stretch. Stand up with your right arm extended above your head. Your palm should be facing the wall. Move your arm slowly down behind you like you are going through the hours, 12 o'clock through 6 o'clock. Repeat with the other arm.

Another helpful stretch if you spend a lot of time at a desk is calf stretches. You can do calf stretches against a wall. Stand on a step and move your heels gently up and down to activate your calf muscles.

HOW TO STRETCH WHILE TRAVELING

Something we do a lot more of (now that we're 50+) is travel – short and long-distance. We've found that traveling by car, plane, or train can put an enormous amount of strain on the body. You end up positioning your body incorrectly, carrying your luggage in all the wrong ways, and slouching. It's not great for your posture. One of our first tips to traveling 50+ers is to invest in a roller bag (with wheels). Also, if you're using a backpack, wear it correctly – that means wearing the back on both shoulders instead of just one. Lastly, make an effort to sit up straight as much as possible – be conscious of it.

Below are a few quick stretches you can do while traveling to give your body and muscles a break - they deserve it.

Upper Back

The tightness can set in quickly in your upper back during travel.

- Place both feet evenly on the floor.
- Lift your arms in front of you, bending them at the elbow.
- Then, cross your arms to clasp your hands together.
- Gradually push your arms away, stretching your back.

Ankles

Ankles have a nasty habit of getting swollen and uncomfortable during long flights. Hydrating is the first step to avoiding this, but there are also some stretches you can do.

- Lift your ankles one at a time and gently roll each ankle to flex and stretch the joint. This action will usually be enough to increase circulation and reduce swelling.
- Repeat the ankle flex every 30 minutes.
- Make sure you get up and move around every 2 hours, whether in a car or a plane.

Neck and Shoulders

You may notice your neck and shoulders are the first to start feeling uncomfortable.

- Place one arm on your seat and the other arm over your shoulder.
- Next, gently pull your head toward the extended arm. This action should stretch your neck and shoulder to loosen stiff muscles.
- Remember to breathe in and out all the way.
- Repeat on the other side.

Hips

The hips can experience discomfort if you have to sit in one position for a long time.

- Lift your right ankle onto your left knee.
- Gently press your knee toward the floor. This will give your right hip a decent stretch.
- Switch to the other leg.

As you can see, there's a stretch for just about every ache, pain, and discomfort. If you want to enjoy a healthy, mobile and independent life, the trick is to stretch every day. Make stretching your "thing."

Armed with all the information you currently have, it's time to move onto Chapter Eight: *How to Stay Healthy Long-Term.*

8

HOW TO STAY HEALTHY LONG TERM

Being 50+ comes with its challenges. You're not as young as you use to be, and often, that thinking takes over. Now that you've got the knowledge and tools for crafting a healthier lifestyle, there's no guarantee that you're going to put it to good used. Just like you might have the recipe for a delicious chocolate cake nobody can say "no" to, you might not make it every weekend. And that's part of the human condition, not the 50+ condition.

Losing your pizazz for something is somewhat normal in life. Ebb and flow in all things are to be expected to some degree, but the trick to ensure that you don't gradually let your newfound health and fitness slip away from you is to strategize for success. Set in place some preventative safeguards for quitting – yup, those are little measures that *don't allow* you to quit.

One of the most effective "safeguards" we have found is to commit ourselves to keep moving. You might not have the inclination to do a full workout every day, but on those days, remember your commitment to move. Do a few stretches that will keep your muscle memory current and your flexibility primed. In the famous Katherine Hepburn's words, "If you don't move, you rust."

Let's take her advice to heart and focus on a few strategies to stay fit and healthy long term and not just for a few weeks. Be cognizant of the fact that your body and mind must serve you well, not just in your 50s, but for the next 10, 20, or even 30 years. That's a lot of mileage your body still has to handle, so you better get a good maintenance plan started *now*. 50 isn't the end of the road! In fact, you're just approaching a bend in the road – so much more awaits you around that bend.

KEEPING YOUR HEAD IN THE GAME

Before we introduce you to a few supplementary materials to help take the stretches and routines you have learned to the next level, we'd like to share a few tips on how to "keep your head in the game" and stay interested in stretching, fitness, and health beyond the pages of this book.

Combine plans with opportunities for fitness.

Combining plans with fitness opportunities is not as strange as you think. We've established that your 50+ body needs to keep moving and that you can't really afford to miss your stretching routines, walks, and healthy food choices. It's easier to incorporate these things into your daily life if you plan to. For instance, if you've got the grand-kids for the day, instead of watching television with them, coloring for hours, or playing card games, start a game of your own where you all have to complete a certain set of activities before presenting everyone with a reward. See where we're going with this? Your stretch routine can be an activity. This way, you're spending quality time with the grandkids while you're getting the movement and stretching you need.

If you want to spend time with your daughter, instead of just heading to the restaurant for brunch, you can meet her in the park for a walk and a homemade fruit smoothie. You will find several ways to combine plans with your loved ones with opportunities for fitness – you just have to give it some thought.

Keep Your Mind Focused on Fitness and Health

By now, you're in your 50s or beyond, and you're well aware of the role the mind plays. No doubt, you have tussled with your mind many times over decisions, scenarios, thoughts, and feelings. The mind is a powerful tool. Once it latches onto an idea, it's hard to get it to let go. You can use this characteristic to your advantage. Expose your mind to more fitness and health-related content and media. The more you see it, read it, watch it, talk about it – the more likely you're going to develop an interest and passion for it. And it's a lot easier to stick to something you're interested in – trust us on that one.

Find Your Health and Fitness Tribe

It's not easy being 50+ and wanting to live a "cleaner" life. Heck, it would have been hard at 30 or 40! The world around you is and will be stuck in its ways. People want to continue being the way they have been for decades – many people don't want change. There's an entire population of 50+ers who would scoff at the idea of getting fit and in shape *now*. Much the same, that population is stuck in a cycle of poor food choices, not enough sleep, over-consumption of alcohol and other bad habits that don't just lead to aches, pains and dependency, but actually shorten their lifespan. That's okay. We want to tell you that you don't have to be like everyone else.

You're well within your rights to take your future into your hands and while there are millions of people in your age group that might go against you, rest assured they're not in *our* club. You just need to find your tribe. Just like there are millions of people out there willing to continue making the unhealthy choices they've been making all along, there are millions of 50+ers who have realized the value in healthy living and staying active. These people are *your* people. Find them and stay close to them!

Where do you find them? The first place to start looking is community fitness groups and health and fitness classes aimed at people 50+. You don't have to join a group or class forever, but you can meet other 50+ers who are in a similar mindset to you by going a few times. Strike up a few friendships because these are the people you can call on for a chat and a walk or a Sunday morning stretch session on the beach.

Another place you can find a support network of active 50+ers is on social media. If you're not on social media, you can ask someone to help you with that, but the chances are that you have *some* presence on the likes of Facebook. Facebook is filled with groups for seniors, and these groups serve as a place for like-minded people to share ideas, provide support, and cheer for each other along the way.

When you feel like you're not alone in it and have others around you or in touch with you working towards similar goals as you, it's easier to stick to the plan - this is another thing you should trust us on.

KNOW YOUR WHY

"Know your why" is something we tell every 50+er we meet who struggles to stick to the plan or only stretch and exercise sporadically. You've undoubtedly spent your life learning about the importance of goal setting, and in your 50s and beyond, goal setting is still important. Having purpose and reasons for doing things isn't a strategy simply for the boardroom – it's a great strategy for life. If you know *why* you want to start stretching and getting fit, you can keep reminding yourself and even use them as motivation along the way.

Many 50+ers have similar reasons for focusing on their physical health, but there will be a few differences here and there. To inspire you to draw up a why-list of your own, we're sharing our reasons below. Perhaps these apply to you too.

- It's fun to play games competitively. We thoroughly enjoy

playing golf, pickleball, tennis, and going for runs with our friends. Without a healthy stretching routine, these activities would be considerably more challenging for us to enjoy.

- No one wants to become a burden on their loved ones. It stands to reason that at some point, our children will take care of us. Talk about turned tables, right? We don't want to become a burden on our children prematurely, if at all. By stretching and maintaining a level of physical fitness, we get to keep our independence.

- To shed the tummy tire. It almost feels like weight finds its way to the midsection the moment you hit your mid-forties, and it just gets worse from there. By staying active, the tummy tire can start to reduce.

- Healthy organs. As we get older, we need to ensure we're doing things that *help* our organs do their job. For instance, IBS is an issue that seems to plague older people. This is when the digestive system and all the organs involved seem to be at some sort of war, and the result is gas, discomfort, pain, and unmentionable bathroom antics. Another problem that can crop up is heart health – cholesterol, high blood pressure – you know how it goes. Stretching and regular exercise can help all manner of problems related to organ health and function. Exercise increases blood flow, thus delivering more healthy oxygen to essential organs – which means your organs get the nourishment they need to function better.

- Mental health boost. Depression, lethargy, sadness, listlessness – none of these sound fun because they're not. Exercise gives you something to focus on other than your mental health problems, and it also inspires a fresh release of feel-good endorphins in the brain that help reduce all of the above-mentioned mental health issues.

- To keep up with the grandkids. If you have grandkids, you already know how high-energy they can be. If you want to keep up with them, you have to maintain a good energy and fitness level. Stretching and exercise is the answer.

Make Stretching and Fitness a Habit

You do several of the same things daily because you have been doing them for years. You have habits, and the sooner you make your fitness routines a habit, the sooner they will become part of daily life. You'll soon start doing them automatically. To develop a healthy habit, you can start by setting reminders. Stick a post-it-note on your fridge to remind you to do 5-10 squats every time you open it. Leave a small set of dumbbells at the front door to inspire a few bicep curls when you enter and leave the house.

Another way to develop a habit is to set reminders on your mobile phone and schedule stretching and workout routines. We find that first thing in the morning is the easiest for us. As we get out of bed, we complete a series of stretches to get the day started. If you have some free time around lunchtime, set a reminder on your phone to spend 15 minutes stretching. Keep setting these reminders until you no longer need them. If you have a favorite television program that runs for around 30 minutes, be ready for it in your workout kit - ready to stretch your way through the episode. Meeting up with a friend regularly for exercise is a great way to develop a habit and stay on track. If you have to meet someone, you become more accountable and more likely to develop a regular habit.

Focus on Rest & Relaxation

Of course, it's not all about exercise. You also need to ensure that your body is getting enough rest and repair so that it can heal and be strong. If you overdo it, your immune system will take a knock, and you will only set yourself back. Because of this, it's important to plan your exercise for the week. Set out the times and days and set the remaining time for rest. During your rest times, make sure you're sleeping enough, eating right, practicing deep breathing (which is great for anxiety and high blood pressure, by the way), and stretching, but in a relaxing way. If you allow your body time to rest, it will serve you even better when you need it to be active and strong. Now that we've got those tips out the way, we'd like to introduce you to some supplementary materials that you can use to boost your routines (and enjoyment).

SUPPLEMENTARY MATERIALS FOR STRETCHING

INVERSION TABLE

The inversion table is a game-changer for people who suffer from back and neck pain. It's a device you lie down on, and then you adjust the table, so you are almost upside down at a 60-degree angle. The theory behind inversion therapy is that the spine has traction while the body's gravity is shifted. This will ease off the pressure on your back. You just have to read the online reviews and talk to people who have used this therapy to realize that inversion therapy is life-changing for people with back pain. Inversion tables are great for:

- Boosting poor circulation
- Reducing chronic lower back pain
- Easing sciatica
- Making scoliosis more manageable

Inversion therapy increases the fluid around the spinal discs while removing waste from the spine, minimizing inflammation, and boosting lower back blood circulation. After just eight weeks of use, you will notice a difference.

Inversion Therapy Risks

You should not use inversion therapy if you have:

- Eye problems (detached retina in particular)
- Bone and joint disorders
- High blood pressure
- Glaucoma
- Ear infection

- Cerebral sclerosis

Also, if you're obese, take blood-clotting medicine, or are pregnant, you should consult with your physician before trying the therapy.

THE FOAM ROLLER

If you think of a foam roller, you probably think of one of those foam pool flotation devices. But the foam roller we are going to explain is a highly recommended stretching and fitness piece of equipment. Foam rollers range in sizes, uses, and price. You can buy them from retail and online stores, and they don't have to be a huge investment. Runners will swear by foam roller use, especially after a race or a long workout. We find them particularly rewarding in the fitness space. Foam rollers increase circulation, improve movement, and are used as a recovery aid for muscles in a fitness routine. Physical therapists often recommend incorporating these rollers in regular workouts. It's great for:

- Improving range of motion
- Decreasing neuromuscular exhaustion
- Minimizing post-exercise soreness
- Decreasing muscle fatigue after an activity
- Increasing muscle performance

A small foam roller is about 5-8 inches in diameter and can target most muscle groups. This is a good size for portability. Also, the firmer the roller, the deeper the pressure you will receive. If you are new to foam rolling, you should start with a softer foam roller.

Foam Rolling Exercises

Calves

To stretch and strengthen your calves: Sit on the floor with your legs extended. Your hands should be on the floor, supporting your body weight. Place the foam roller under both calves and then rest the right ankle on the left leg. Slowly roll the roller along the back of the left leg from the knee to the ankles. Repeat for the other leg.

This will lengthen the calf muscle and help prevent ankle stiffness. This is helpful early in the day, after a workout, or if you sit all day.

Quads

To use the foam roller for your quads:

Lie face-down on the floor and place the foam roller under your upper legs. Roll up and down from your hips to your knees.

If you are a cyclist or a runner, you will find this most useful. Foam rolling the quads will help improve flexibility in the knee, reduce tension in your upper leg, and increase mobility in your hips. This stretch with the foam roller will benefit you before a bike ride or a run by increasing the ease of mobility. Use it after a workout to decrease soreness.

Hamstrings

Sit with your left leg on the foam roller. Bend your left knee and then place your hands behind you for balance. Start rolling up and then down from your knee to right under your hips. Then switch legs.

This will loosen your upper leg, improve hip mobility, and decrease stress on your back. This will help soreness after a workout and also help you stretch if you sit at a desk all day.

Outer Thighs

Lie on your left side with the foam roller under your left hip. Your left leg should extend fully out. Place your left hand extended to the floor. Your right leg is bent over your left leg with your right foot on the floor for balance. Roll up and back on your left thigh. Repeat on the other side.

This is particularly important for women to do because of anatomical differences between women and men. Women have tighter outer thighs than men. Rolling this area can decrease stress on both the hips and the knees.

Back

Sit down on the ground with the foam roller positioned under your lower back. Lock your fingers behind your head and bend your knees. Use your knees to push yourself over the roller - up and down your back to right below your shoulder blades and back to your lower back again.

Using the foam roller on your back will help relieve tightness and improve muscle activation. Rolling under your back is a good stretch any time of the day to decrease stiffness.

Shoulders and Sides

Lie down on your left side, with the foam roller under the left side of your chest with your left arm extended out on the floor away from your torso. Your left leg should be straight on the ground, and your right leg should be propped in front of your body with the knee bent. Move slowly up and down on the roller, so the left side and lower shoulder contact the roller. Then, move toward the legs.

Buttocks

Sit on the foam roller and cross the left leg over the right knee. Lean toward the left hip and put your weight on your right hand for support. Slowly roll over the right cheek and then switch sides.

Your glutes are the most extensive muscle group in your body. Working on the glutes is a great stretch to do before climbing stairs, running or cycling. A good time to stretch the glutes is after desk sitting or a tough workout.

EXERCISE BALL

An exercise ball is a popular stretching tool for all age groups. Used both in physical rehab for healing and in classrooms worldwide for core workouts while sitting, the exercise ball is a critical tool. We are including the exercise ball in our supplemental stretching tools because you can do so many stretches with this supportive device. Buy a ball that feels comfortable to sit on without the fear of falling or wobbling off. Here are just a few.

Lunge Stretch

Sit on your exercise ball in a lunge position. Your right leg should be in front, curved around the ball, and your left leg behind. You must be able to rest comfortably on the ball. Bring your arms in front of you and then stretch them overhead. Hold for 3-5 seconds. You will feel a stretch in both your hips and your upper body. Switch to the other leg and repeat. If you feel at all wobbly, make sure you stabilize the ball.

Back Stretch

Stand with the ball in front of you and then bend at the hips so your left forearm touches the ball. Move the ball forward to feel the stretch in the back and hold for 3-5 seconds. Then switch with to your right arm. This is to help release tension in your back.

RESISTANCE BANDS

Resistance or stretch bands help stretch and extend muscles and can take the place of lifting weights. Depending on the thickness of the bands, you can pull up and down with your arms to strengthen shoulder and arm muscles. You can use the resistance band for a full-body workout divided over several days.

Try this one: Stand on the band with your feet shoulder-width apart. Hold the other ends at your sides - have each palm facing away from you. Sit down again into a squat. Push down into your heels and push into a standing position, and as you come to full extension at the knee, curl the handles up toward your shoulders. The more you hold under your foot or in your hand, the more intense the lift and resistance.

These supplemental stretching materials help change up your routines and work on deeper muscle relaxation and tension release. Whether you are experiencing pain in larger muscle groups or smaller, more concentrated groups, these items get your muscles loose and prepared for activity and decrease impact after a hard workout.

We're almost at the point where we pat you on the back and send you out into the world to handle your stretching and fitness on your own. You've gathered all the information and advice you need, and now you have the book with its recommended stretches and routines to refer to as needed.

But before you go, we'd like to end things off with a few words - page over to the final section *Conclusion*.

CONCLUSION

While this is the final page of our Life After 50 *Stretching* book, it's not the end. This is the start of an entirely new chapter. When you turn this page and close this book, you'll already be a new version of yourself, even if you haven't practiced a single stretch yet. Why? Because now you know better. You've expanded your mind and now know just how important it is to stretch and regularly move, not just for you but for your loved ones too. We've spoken about it all in the past eight chapters! We've covered aging, and its impact on flexibility, the benefits of stretching (there are many), and even discussed the common 50+er's range of aches and pains and how to eliminate them.

We then moved on to the types of stretches you should be doing, touched on what "active living" means for someone 50+, and presented you with a wide range of stretches to try. All the stretches included are designed to make everyday activities like gardening, playing golf, reaching for something, or carrying a grandchild easier. Lastly, we presented you with several stretching routines to try and a collection of tips on how to keep it up - and here we are – at the precipice of great things. Those great things are: you taking control of your physical fitness and taking the steps required, or should we say stretches required, to get yourself into the best shape of your 50+ life. By now, you know that stretching:

- Builds muscle strength
- Boosts circulation
- Improves flexibility
- Enhances mobility
- Minimizes aches and pains
- Releases feel-good hormones
- Increases energy levels
- Sheds excess weight
- Balances hormones
- Improves posture
- Boosts organ health and functionality
- Eases aches and pains (especially in joints and muscles)

In short, stretching re-establishes that zest for life that has been slowly fading from you over the years. It puts a pep in your step. It brings about the type of change that has your grandkids saying things like, "What happened to grandad – he's looking so good!" or "I can't wait to see grandma; she's so much fun these days!" Stretching brings back a youthful and vibrant element right back into you, and guess what; you deserve every bit of it!

50+ isn't a time to say that you've done all the living you need to do. It's not the gateway to a series of long and dark years filled with pains, aches, stiffness, and deterioration. It's a time to recalibrate. You can look around you at all you have achieved and all the fun you've had, and then take a deep breath (and a stretch) and say, "Here's to the next 50!" because with stretching and keeping active, you could very well have 50 more years ahead of you.

With all of this said, we'd love to extend a heartfelt thank you to everyone who took the time to read our book and learn about the possibilities of a healthy, active, and rewarding life after crossing the border of 50. We'd love to keep producing content like this to help other 50+ers make a positive change in their lives. If you liked our book, we would appreciate an honest review on Amazon (thanks in advance!).

In health and fitness in the 50+ club together,

Alicia Diaz and Lee Davidson.

Additional Sources Used

- Frutel, Natasha. 2019. Reviewed by Dr. Peggy Pilcher. M.S. R.D. L.D. CDE. *Stretching Exercises to Improve Mobility for Seniors.* Retrived on 5/07/2021 from https://www.healthline.com/health/senior-health/stretching-exercises
- Hamilton, Michelle. 2021. *How to Use a Foam Roller. Retrieved* on 06/05/2021 from: https://www.runnersworld.com/health-injuries/a20812623/how-to-use-a-foam-roller-0/
- Mansour, Stephanie. 2019/updated 2021. *The Best Resistant Bands of 2021- and a 30-Day Work Out Plan to Put Them to Work.* Retrieved on 6/01/2021 from: https://www.nbcnews.com/better/lifestyle/one-month-resistance-band-workout-you-can-do-anywhere-ncna965461
- Staff. 2015. *Using Relaxing Techniques to Improve the Health of Older Adults.* Retrieved on 6/01/2021 from: https://careandcomfortathome.com/using-relaxation-techniques-to-improve-the-health-of-older-adults/
- Blackwell, Rebecca. 2020. *Why Stretching is Important In Active and Aging Seniors.* retrieved on 05/07/2021 from: Ahttps://blog.hurusa.com/why-stretching-is-important-in-active-aging-and-functional-training

Just For You!

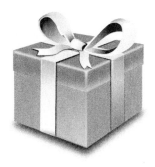

A FREE GIFT TO OUR READERS
Claim Your Gift At:

www.healthylifeafter50.com

Printed in Great Britain
by Amazon

81453851R00129